To Andrena,
It's been a pleasure to meet
you! We did tha kona! pins
and all...

To ___, it ___
prince@gis.net

6/25/01

T5-BQB-721

Teaching
Me to Run

Teaching Me to Run

Tommye-K. Mayer

Prince-Gallison Press Boston, MA 02113

Teaching Me to Run

Prince-Gallison Press, 2001

For information:

Prince-Gallison Press
P.O. Box 23, Hanover Station
Boston, MA 02113-0001
(tel) 617-367-5815
(fax) 617-367-3337

Library of Congress Catalog Card Number 99-90861

ISBN 0-9652805-2-7
Published in the United States
        PRINTED IN THE UNITED STATES OF AMERICA

Dedicated to Dad and Mom, and to everyone who patiently or impatiently listened to me figure out how to teach myself to run—not once, but twice.

Thank you

Also by
Tommye-K. Mayer

"Tommye-K. Mayer is also the author of *"One-Handed in a Two-Handed World."* Described by the editors of OT Week as a self-help book par excellence, *"One-Handed in a Two-Handed World."* is the step-by-step guide to managing just about everything with the use of one hand.

While *"One-Handed in a Two-Handed World."* was written by a stroke survivor, this book is equally applicable to individuals struggling to manage single-handedly as a result of a short-term injury such as rotator cuff injury, broken,bones as well as strains and sprains.

Teaching Me to run is highly recommended by doctors and rehabilitation professionals internationally.

Epigraph

"She had devastating damage to the brain. She was always very motivated, but I didn't think she'd ever be able to do this running. She very pleasantly did not confirm my prognosis."

—Dr. Albert Goodgold, New York University Medical Center, neurologist

Quoted in the Boston Tab, "*One Step at a Time: Stroke survivor overcomes disabilities,*" November 12, 1991

Table of Contents

One:
That intrinsic Joy

IN MID-SENTENCE HE STEPPED AWAY FROM ME, DEEPER into the center of my living room, not focused so much on the movement as on his thought and the words he'd chosen to express it. I'm not sure he was even aware he'd moved.

Me? I was watching as much as listening. Watching and noticing.

It was different now, the way he moved—smooth, more fluid, more confident. It was almost as if, after thirty-five years of living in his body, he'd discovered its extent, and understood that extent now too; understanding the parameters of its parts, internalizing as well, the purposes for each of those parts. It was as if before, his body had been only packaging for his brain, unworthy of his consideration as long as it continued to get what his brain needed and to move his brain where it needed to be.

"It's strange, you know," he was saying, "most of the time I really hate running. I have to make myself get out there and do it."

He stepped, closer to me. I'd begun serving dinner, ziti heaped with steaming hot eggplant stew, one plate already on the table.

"When I was a little kid," he said speaking softly, "if we were thinking about going out just to exercise, my father would tell us to get out the lawn mower or do something con-structive—wash the cars, work out back —so it's strange . . . to be just running." He pursed his lips in a tight smile, eye-brows raised. "Sometimes," he continued, then correcting himself, "—and it happens a lot, as I'm getting to the end of my route, I feel as though I could go on running forever—my legs working, my arms pumping, my heart pounding . . . "

He clenched his hands waist-high, shoulders square, and showed me, jogging only his upper body—his feet unmoving, his cautious, tight-lipped smile shrouded behind his beard.

"I remember," I murmured.

And I did. I remembered running—on hard-packed sand, across grassy playing fields, over red North Carolina dirt, along deep Florida sand, around the Wheaton Dimple, in Central Park, running and laughing between the bases in a spirited game of "pickle," with and playfully away from

2

schoolgirl boyfriends. In that moment, I remembered the feeling of my body running anywhere. Running wherever and whenever I chose to take it.

But especially I remembered running on the beach, on the hard-packed, sandy beach at low-tide in front of my folks' house. Even after ten years, sometimes I still dreamt . . . "What do you suppose it is?" David asked.

We sat down to eat. And to talk more.

"It," I said, dragging myself from my reverie, trying to recall his last remark, and then remembering. "The feeling you could go on forever?"

"Yes," he said, the next forkful poised to eat. "I couldn't, of course. There's a limit to how far the human body can run before it wears out."

I nodded, thinking. "I wonder," I paused, an explanation formulating in my mind, "don't you think feeling you could go on forever has everything to do with the intrinsic joy of a body doing exactly what it's designed to do?"

"What's that?" David asked, deep creases between his eyebrows, at the bridge of his nose, another forkful of pasta suspended between the plate and his mouth.

"Move." As I spoke the one word a wave of sadness passed over me. Only fleetingly— after ten years, the sadness rarely swept as it had once. I'd almost gotten used to limits on my abilities—the physical and those few hidden limits— though I'd never stopped picking away at those limits. I was still "rehabilitating" myself—still punching the envelope of ability despite disability.

"Rehab" was what they'd called it in the hospital —after all these years, I kew it as my life. Two, three hours I worked each afternoon—stretching, strengthening, and on fine movement patterning-type exercises and activities making up a well-rounded physical therapy regimen.

This talk about running had raised an old memory: racing down the middle of the field chasing an unguarded ball, my hockey stick loosely cradled in both hands, parallel to the ground and suspended at mid-thigh, my one-size-fits-all shin pads rubbing their many folds against my ankles, the rubber cleats gripping the turf, my toes pulling, propelling me forward, the muscles in my calves, my thighs, my buttocks, my feet straining.

I remembered picturing, as I ran, a long-legged gazelle bounding gracefully over a field of tall grass, not the elephant on stiletto heels I see in my mind's eye now.

"Hmm," David remarked, interrupting my recollection of my fourteen-year-old self—my thick, mahogany-brown braid slapping the hollow of my spine as I raced after the white, rock-hard and fist-sized field-hockey ball. "That's an interesting idea. I'll have to think about that," he finished.

Even as David and I talked long after dinner, in the back of my mind I remembered how the air burned in my lungs, almost feeling it. Long after school closed, in the late Autumn, toward the end of the game, the sun shining between barren tree branches, the cold air chilling our bare legs, we'd run up and down the field too many times to count.

I AWOKE TO MY ALARM THE NEXT MORNING ONLY VAGUELY aware of a dream about running the beach in front of my parents' home. Twisting the hot and cold handles to the shower one at a time and adjusting the temperature, I thought about how much I'd love to be a fly on the wall for one of David's toward-the-end-of-the-route moments, wondering how else I could actually see him feeling as though he could go on running forever, this man who, for as long as I'd known him, had eschewed exercise of any kind. Or see him even wanting to go on running forever.

But better than that, the thought seized me: What if I could do it myself? What if I could run again?

TWO:
What if

HOW LONG DID I STAND UNDER THE WATER FLOW, LOST in the idea and all the while thinking *but how?* Mechanically, I squeezed shampoo along my hairline the way I always did before rubbing it into my hair, thinking: about the ten years half my body had been partially paralyzed—hemi-paresis they call it.

I couldn't even imagine any more how a body runs. I stood, the hot water cooling to lukewarm as I rinsed the shampoo from my hair. Even walking my best, my left leg still felt, "like light looks through water," as I'd described it to the physical therapist on my first day of physical therapy in the rehabilitation hospital. Sitting with me on the exercise table, he'd asked what a paralyzed leg felt like.

And yet, quickly my "impetuous imp" side grew enthusiastic as the questions came: What was running? How did it work? What did it look like? What did it feel like? The questions terrifying as much as intriguing me as the water pelting my body cooled more. Pretty soon it'd be ice cold, and yet my imp side had me trying to march in place, the water pouring over me. My right foot and leg stepped smartly. But the left—even though she walked sort of okay, with only a bit of a limp—raised hesitantly and clumsily, as if instructions from my mind to my leg were passing through distant or poorly spliced connections.

PULLING ON CLOTHES, I THOUGHT ABOUT HOW TEN years after fifty cc's of blood had flooded the thalamic region of my brain—I could now walk as far as I wanted, with only a hitch to my step. I was supposed to live my life from a wheelchair, and then, never capable of leaving behind the leg brace and cane. So wasn't walking reasonably well, as much as I could hope for? I'd recovered a darn sight more than their predictions for me—way more. So wasn't I just troubling trouble with these thoughts of running?

The imp in me chimed in: Is it as much as you could do? It's always been my imp, the overly optimistic, fun-focused child inside me that's pushed me to try—to try walking without the cane and then without the brace, to try figuring out how to manage just about everything single-handedly, to try—just eighteen months after the hemorrhage—to get back on skis, even bashing more than a few of Breckenridge's black-diamond mogul fields with the New England Handicapped Sports Association, until some guy cut across the tips of my boards, taking my left ski with him and tearing a ligament in my vulnerable left knee.

What if I could run.

I set my coffee on the table. The whole thing was ridiculous. I pulled my bagel out of the toaster oven and glanced at the telephone. No, David wouldn't call this morning—he was just here last night. It'd be tomorrow or the next day before I heard from him again—he was like that.

Was he out running right now? In the periphery of my attention I noticed the time. Geez! I grabbed my stuff and the rest of my bagel, heading for the door. Walking the half mile to catch the shuttle van near Boston's North Station to take me out to the World Trade Center, I chewed on my bagel, still trying to imagine David running.

I climbed into the front seat of the van I rode every morning, digging the fingers of my one hand into the gutter over the door, my right foot on the step plate. Between my right arm and leg, I hiked my torso high and twisted, lowering my buttocks onto the seat, then released my grip on the gutter and closed the door behind me. I always tried to be the first in the van. Getting into the back bench seats was far more complicated.

I still thought about running, still remembered doing it,

and still I wondered, How does it work? How does a person run? Outside the window, a flood of commuters pushed through the doors, gushing out of North Station, hurrying across in front of the van.

A train must have just pulled in, delivering these hundreds of commuters to the city from the northern suburbs, all thronging from within the building onto Causeway Street to make their way downtown to the financial district. Each individual moved purposefully, some clutching briefcases, arms swinging. They all moved swiftly—but still walked.

I studied their movements, noticing individual variations, the different twists each had added to the basic act of walking, trying to understand the differences.

Since the hemorrhage, I'd watched so many people walk—studying the hows, the whats, and the whys of walking. Over the years. I'd tried to internalize how a person accomplished the special fluidity I now saw again. What exactly was she doing? What muscles was he using? Why did this or that part of her body also move when she walked? How did men and women do it differently?

This time, as I studied, I found myself trying to understand what would be different if the people were running instead of walking. They kept coming out of the station, trainload after trainload. I concentrated on my study, not noticing other passengers pulling open the sliding door behind me, and boarding the van.

It was late August—cooler than the heat of summer but

not yet jacket weather. Even though the people I watched were dressed for the office, they wore lightweight clothing, allowing me to follow their movements. I kept watching, even as Paul shifted the transmission from Park into Drive. Once we got to the World Trade Center, I'd be in cubicle village for the next eight and a half hours, with no more opportunity to study anything but the text and digits on my computer screen.

Maybe I'd get over this new fixation on running, this wondering if somehow I could figure out how I could run. Surely me, "running" was an absolutely ridiculous idea. After all, I was the one who wasn't supposed to survive half a cup of blood cascading into the thalamic region of my brain. And when I did, they worried maybe I shouldn't have. The devastating damage to my brain should have made me a vegetable. They expected I'd never step out of a wheelchair—or get into one unassisted.

But that was while I was still in intensive care. Once I'd awakened from the coma and was transferred to the rehabilitation hospital, it was clear I would walk. Of course, when the rehabilitation hospital released me, I wore a steel-and-leather "single-action" leg brace attached to heavy, flexible steel-shank shoes, relied on a straight cane, and only sort of walked—straight-kneed, like a tin soldier.

After a while, working on my own, I no longer relied on the cane to walk and then shed the leg brace and those godawful shoes, learning to bend my left knee with each step. I had only a bit of a limp, and I could walk as far as I wanted (except on smooth linoleum or marble floors, where I still tended to catch my toe, because my foot didn't automatically pick up at the ankle when I raised my left leg with each step —something to do with my dorsi flexion and plantar flexion, resulting in what my physical therapist called "drop-foot"). So the toe on my left shoe sometimes got scuffed scraping against pavement underfoot. It was really only a problem when the toe of my rubber-soled left shoe rubbed against, sort of sticking to, linoleum floors or highly finished wood floors.

As we drove up the ramp to the World Trade Center, I found myself acknowledging a history usually appreciated only by others looking in on my life—the history of how much progress I'd made since I was twenty-three years, two months, and a few days old, awakening from a coma.

It was different, looking at my life from the outside. Typically I'd focused on how much I'd lost and not on how much I'd regained. Well, I thought, at the risk of getting a fat head, maybe it was time to reframe.

Three:
What Running Is

LIFE WENT ON, BUT STILL THE IDEA OF TEACHING MYSELF to run hovered over everything, bubbling in the back of my mind. My life was full already—working full-time, friends, dating, and the hours of maintenance physical therapy I did each day since leaving the rehabilitation hospital in 1981; patterning exercises, stretching, strengthening, and half an hour pushing hard on my rowing machine.

Over and over, I'd find myself deeply lapsed into ruminations about the hows of running, anywhere—in line at the bank, at the market, in the cafeteria, sitting in Keith's swivel chair wrapped in a purple smock when he'd fallen silent as he cut my hair, waiting for the van, a bus, the subway, during lapses in conversation, walking—even just around the corner.

The pull to run again was so strong. I attended to it, studying my memory of it, as if the images in my mind were an opposing team's video you watch over and over. In my mind eye, I'd replay runners I'd seen, close-focusing on segments of their running—sometimes studying only feet, only knees, or perhaps only shoulders, just trying to understand.

So hmm, I'd think, how would it work for me? the grownup voice in my mind would ask as I became aware of my thoughts, the images so vivid sometimes I'd feel it, sometimes I'd swear I could feel again the breeze of my own making brushing past my face, blowing through my hair. And sometimes I'd even feel the thick braid I used to wear thwacking one-two, one-two, against my spine with each stride.

It was gone, long gone, that waist-length hair, gone since just days, or perhaps just hours, following the bleed—though still I could feel it in my memory. I'd feel the pounding through my bones, all the way up, from my feet to my head. I'd feel the straining in my muscles throughout, my ligaments, my tendons. I'd feel the need in my lungs to draw in more air than just staying-alive breathing.

Each time I caught my mind straying into such dangerous territory, I'd veer away, distracting myself, substituting some other thought, maybe focusing on the juxtaposition of historic architecture with I. M. Pei–like glass and steel, noticing a particularly interesting face, hearing a snatch of conversation, refocusing on the book I intended to be reading, the music in the background.

It was dangerous territory because of how much I still wanted it all back—all the ability I'd lost to the hemorrhage—

and, in failing to get it all, how hard I continued working at it. And dangerous because of how much the running had come to symbolize to me.

Whenever thoughts of running filled my mind, anticipation surged through my body, from the soles of my feet, up, up, through my spine—an electricity rising up the back of my neck and all through my scalp. I recognized, that feeling—an anticipation I'd once known so well, the heightened expectancy that almost had a flavor, that set in before a competition when I'd felt as prepared as I would ever be and finally it was nearly time to prove it. The electricity that ended up churning in my stomach masquerading as nausea, sort of.

It terrified the grownup in me to want so much, when so very possibly, perhaps even probably, what I wanted would end in defeat and maybe even physical damage. So much of me counseled Maybe it would be better to leave it alone. Wouldn't it be safer to just walk away from what must surely lead to failure?

Failing would be too difficult, confronting me all over again with how much I, the girl whose pediatrician once described as having "the best muscular-skeletal development of any child he'd ever seen," had really lost. Forcing me to face all over again how much I couldn't do anymore. By trying to run, I risked showing myself once more what used to be and couldn't be anymore, I risked overwhelming myself with the devastation again.

So much of me argued the wisdom of shutting down desires like this, reasoned for continuing as I was, for being satisfied with what I had. Hadn't I worked hard enough for what I was able to do now—so much of it bought with my own sweat, blood, and probably even pounds of my own flesh? I'd forever wear the scars from the countless cuts and scrapes gained by pushing myself beyond Dr. Goodgold's prognosis.

I was thirty-two years old. Already, it was nine years since the hemorrhage. Wasn't time to tell myself Tomm, you don't need to keep pushing so hard. It's not necessary to keep pushing the envelope so you're left picking yourself up off the pavement when you crash. Take a rest, kick back, pat yourself for the job you've done already. It's enough. Hon, already you almost pass for normal. Can't you be okay with that?

So much of me wanted to be able to quit the constant push to rehabilitate. So much argued it was time to shift my focus in other directions—maybe try accomplishing important, change-the-world things, maybe try living a "normal person's" life, doing "normal" things. Maybe a career change, maybe writing novels, maybe love, marriage, and even a family. "Normal" people did plenty of interesting things . . .

But isn't running something "normal" people do? the imp in me piped up, and my grown-up mind shuddered, because Oh, the dreams . . . . Grown-up me was responsible for protecting and taking care of the playful, optimistic, "What if?" imp that was me too. How could I even attempt to accomplish "normal" things if I damaged myself attempting what I had no business trying? the grown-up reasoned.

So much of me wanted to throw out what threatened to evolve into a goal and a passion called "What-If-I-Could-Run-Again," wanted to ignore this longing to be able to move faster than always walking, to forget the desire to feel a breeze from my own movement against my face, lifting the bangs off my forehead. The need to be completely "normal" again and do "normal" things again, to be part of the group again, in a way other than just a talking head with good ideas.

And yet, in the scheme of things, weren't there other, more sensible ways to do it? What, after all would being able to run do for me?

Well.., the imp in me jumped in to respond. It's the imp that has pushed me beyond reasonable expectations and punched the envelope beyond recognition. If you could run, it would be fun. The imp was jumping up and down urging.

Even responsible me was attracted to the prospect of "fun." And if you could run, it would feel good. If you could run, you could do more stuff with other people, the imp continued building the momentum. If you could run, you could participate, instead of only spectating. If you could run, maybe you'd move better, too—more fluidly, less awkwardly. . . more "normal." If you could run, any number of opportunities might open up . . . you just never know. But most of all— most of all—it would be fun.

As dangerous as it was to think about, let alone actually try, that impish voice was noisy. And the lure of fun became irresistible. How do you fight "fun" when so much of life post-cerebral-hemorrhage, is decidedly unfun?

"IF YOU KNOW WHAT YOU WANT TO DO, YOU CAN DO what you want," Moshe Feldenkrais said. Feldenkrais, a

Russian-Israeli mechanical engineer, developed a mind-body alternative therapy at first to resolve painful, crippling—and, for Western medicine, irreparable—soccer damage to his knees. Over time, Feldenkrais had become unable to walk. Applying his mechanical-engineering background to his body, Feldenkrais developed a mind-body philosophy and taught himself to do the "impossible," he "taught" himself to walk again.

Since the summer of 1982, which I'd spent at a Feldenkrais training at Hampshire College learning the Method as a practice subject for teachers and trainees, the Feldenkrais Method had became an integral part of my ongoing rehabilitation. The Method reinforced the way I'd intuitively studied how able-bodied people move, and broken down movement into manageable parts, and saw the whole as more than, while still, the sum of its parts.

I'd been watching TABs (the Temporarily Able-Bodied people) in motion before I found Feldenkrais. But Feldenkrais had validated and reinforced my own ideas about knowing "normal" movement by watching it, and understanding each movement by reducing it to its parts and then learning to copy.

So, if I planned to actually teach myself to run, I had to figure out what, exactly, running was. I needed to know, intellectually emotionally, and physiologically—in my bones and in my muscles, what TABs do when they run. I needed to know what I had done automatically when I'd run almost ten years ago.

I had to know what it would feel like inside—in my bones,

in my muscles, and in my tendons and ligaments—to run. How it would work. I needed to watch running. I needed to study it. Where did people go to run? I thought about the Esplanade—I'd heard talk about running beside the Charles River—but by the time I got there after work, the sun would be setting. How could I see the detail I needed?

After work, I settled into a park bench beside the HarborWalk near the Marriott Long Wharf Hotel, and there they were—runners of all shapes and sizes and abilities. Day after day, after work I'd bring a little something for supper down to the HarborWalk, settle in, and watch until it got too dark, and the mosquitoes began eating me alive. I'd study thirty-somethings—like me—only running. I'd watch children, I'd study twenty-somethings, and I watched folks much older, but still running.

And I analyzed what I saw, trying to figure out how the ones who ran well moved so fluidly, so smoothly. I also studied less athletic runners, comparing them to the others. What made the difference? Was it power, strength, coordination— or was it simply practice? Or perhaps the difference was an instinctive knowledge, an innate perception athletes have about their bodies that lesser runners just don't? I watched the less skilled runners, because it seemed as important to understand what didn't work as to understand a smooth stride and graceful form.

Mostly I watched the runners who made running look effortless, watching their feet, their legs, their upper bodies, their shoulders, their arms, necks, even their heads. I studied everything, each element of their bodies individually, as a part of the whole, and the whole, seeking all the while to figure out how they did it—what made their movement so fluid?

And I worked on bringing back my body memories, on trying to remember its feeling fluid and natural once, though I still didn't know how I'd done it—just that I had. Watching, I wondered if it had looked as fluid when I'd run. Was I ever a smooth, strong runner? Perhaps, I thought. Perhaps before the AVM, the congenital defect in my cerebral circulatory system that caused the hemorrhage, began interfering with my coordination. Listening to the labored breathing of one runner at the end of her run, I almost felt the burning pressure in my own chest, remembering.

The late summer warmth allowed my running subjects to bare much of their bodies As they ran by, I could see the muscles they used. The shorts and tank tops allowed me to study nearly whole bodies of the few lean, muscular "real" runners. Nearly whole bodies—all but their feet.

As for feet, I had to extrapolate, based on how each shoe struck the pavement, interpreting how the bones, muscles, tendons, and ligaments worked, imagining the gimballing in the ankle, the bend at the toes. Listening to the sound of feet landing on pavement, I got clues to how running is supposed to happen.

Sometimes while watching the runners, I'd untie and take off my shoe and, slipping off my sock, I'd manipulate the toes and ankle of my left foot, feeling the flex of the joints, reminding each how it could move, showing how it would move when I ran. Once I understood what was supposed to happen, the trick would be figuring out how, using what movement I had, to do what I wanted.

Four:
Not just, like walking fast?

DAVID AND I HURRIED, WALKING AS FAST AS I COULD. If we were lucky, we'd make the seven o'clock showing of *Prince of Tides* at the Charles Cinema. Passing the Boston Garden, I struggled to keep up, still insisting it wasn't a problem. When we'd first gotten together that evening, David had marveled at how much more energy he seemed to have, now that he was running.

"I do some work until lunch or so, go for a run, and then, you know, shower and change, and I can finish up a whole other day's work."

Watching me trip, just barely catching myself while trying to keep up and talk at the same time, David didn't miss a step pulling open the rear side door of a taxicab idling at the stand beside the curb.

"Come on, Tommye, let's take a cab," he said, waiting for me to step in.

"All right, but would you get in first? It's hard to lift my left leg over the hump that's the driveshaft," I said, a smile on my lips, laughter sneaking out with the words. Telling him, telling anyone what I had trouble with shamed me.

David shrugged, then lowered himself into the cab, onto the back seat, somewhat awkwardly arranging his broad-shouldered frame into the space behind the driver. As we drove away from the curb, the driver muttering about the unprofitably short fare, I responded to the question David had asked, the question I'd been thinking about when I caught my toe and nearly landed face-first on the pavement. I'd just told him I was thinking about teaching myself to run.

Furrowing his brow, his lips a thin white-red line, he'd asked, "What's to teach? Isn't it just like walking extra fast?"

"Actually," I replied, my shoulders turned to face him, "running is very different from walking, from walking fast, or even from race walking. I've been studying walking and running both."

"So, what's the difference?"

I pressed my lips together, planning the words I needed to explain it clearly. "If you concentrate on how it feels when you're out running next time, you'll sense there's a moment in each stride when you're airborne—a moment when no part of either foot is touching the ground. That's the difference—the airborneness."

I noticed the taxi driver, a guy twenty or so years older than I, nodding silently. He hadn't joined our conversation, so maybe he wasn't even listening . . .

David, his eyes locked on mine, the vertical lines between his eyebrows deeply creased, frowned, "So what's involved in teaching yourself to run?"

"I'm not sure." I paused. "But I think finding the right place to do it is the critical first step."

"Tell me about the right place. What does it look like?"

The taxi had turned into the parking lot for the theater and was pulling up to the curb. I would be the first one out. As I reached for the door handle, before pulling, I glanced at David "I don't know," I admitted.

It was a second-floor theater, accessed either by stairs or a ramp zigzagging up a gentle grade. I paused beside the cab, waiting for David to get out. Something about his question had me looking at the ramp.

It wasn't much to look at—just a run-of-the-mill, utilitarian, steel-and-cement urban construction, but on top of David's question, it got me thinking.

"Shall we take the ramp or the stairs?" he asked.

"The stairs." Between my strong arm and leg, I'd learned

to climb stairs much faster than following the serpentined ramp path.

"Okay, let's go."

Grabbing the steel-pipe railing, I stepped onto the first tread with my right foot, drawing my left leg over the next tread and onto the next. Pulling with my arm, I brought my weaker leg over the next tread, then still up and over and onto the next with my strong leg, clearing two steps at a time.

The railing was central. It allowed me to take the chance—to push two stairs with each stride. Nearing the top, I glanced through the glass partition separating the stairs from the ramp for this last bit of the climb. It was a gentle slope, complying with the Commonwealth's Architectural Barriers codes. The same steel-pipe railing lined both side walls of the ramp at about waist height.

This might not be an appropriate place. But what if? I found myself thinking, the germ of an idea forming: a handrail, or something my one hand could rest against and use to help out in case I fell. That might enable me to break through what at that moment I now knew as the fear barrier, the barrier to learning to run because of the fear of falling and the fear of being airborne for that moment at each running step.

Five:
The Shoes

Someone had propped open the front door to the neighborhood storefront sports shop. I stepped inside and recognized the smell right away: new leather-and-rubber athletic shoes, iron-on team-jersey appliqué adhesive, old wooden floors, the balls—basketball soccer, baseball, football—each with its own smell, the hockey pucks, sticks, and skates, and, of course, the old equipment and an ever-present, lingering sweat. All familiar smells to me, though I still felt out of place. What if it were ridiculous for a stroke survivor to talk about learning to run, what if someone laughed?

"Can I help you?" He was alone, cashing out the register? I wondered. On the wall behind, an old Coca-Cola clock showed a quarter to five. Pushing the register drawer shut he made his way around the counter toward me.

I'd seen this guy before. Where? maybe coaching one of the neighborhood softball teams? He seemed friendly, about my height, somewhere around my age, dark hair, and white, white teeth. He smiled broadly—completely nonthreatening. In red script, I read his name, "Ted" stitched on the pocket of his team jersey.

"Ah," I said, pausing. "Yeah, I'm here for a pair of running shoes."

Was it my imagination, or did I see him raise his eyebrows? Somewhat skeptical, perhaps? Embarrassed, I laughed through my nose and then finished with, "I'm going to teach myself to run."

"Okay." It didn't seem to faze him. His only question; "What size are you?" Rapidly pulling three shoe boxes from among the stacks along the wall, he turned to me saying, "Sit down, try these."

I sat down untying my left shoe and loosening the lace to take it off. Trying on shoes always felt awkward. Over the years, I'd reduced the process to fitting my paralyzed foot. If that shoe fit, the right shoe probably would.

Ted watched me put my left foot into all three left shoes. Somehow, the second felt better. Of course, the shoes were laced normally—not manageable with one hand. I'd re-lace the pair I bought for one-handed tying once I got home. Years ago I'd discovered I could just pull regularly laced laces tight and then stuff the ends into the shoe just below my ankle bones when I wanted to walk in the shoes I was trying on.

As I began stuffing one end of the lace, Ted asked, "You want me to tie that? I see you have your own way. . . but why don't I do these, just to try them?"

He crouched down, squatting in front of my foot and adjusted the laces over the tongue before tying a firm bow. Then he reached into the box, taking out the other shoe.

"You've got to try them both on and walk around some. I'll tie this one too." He never spoke the dreaded "for you," an unnecessary phrase that served only to point out to me yet another thing people noticed I didn't do as well now.

With both shoes on, I stood and stepped the few paces across the room, then around the clothes rack and back. Of course Ted watched, and of course "the kids" (my left arm and leg, because they act like two two-year-old children permanently attached to my body) weren't behaving—spastic tone in my calf and hamstrings made the knee even less fluid, the ankle wobbly, and my elbow tighten into a firm right angle sticking out to the side, my fingers clenched in a fist. He must think I should save my money, I thought, but instead, I said, "These 'sneakers' feel great." I laughed, laughing because somehow I knew they didn't call them sneakers any more, because the running shoes really did feel good on my feet, and because "the kids" were acting so embarrassingly crippled. "With these," I waved my hand toward the floor, indicating the shoes, "I might actually be able to do this."

That was when Ted asked what had happened to me. It was okay now, since he'd become a co-conspirator in my running project. That gave him a right to know.

"So how do you teach yourself to run?" he asked.

"I'm not exactly sure," I looked at him, my eyebrows disappearing under my bangs. "It sort of sounds to you like teaching yourself to do something like swallowing, doesn't it?" I laughed, scrunching my lips toward my nose.

"Well. . . ." He nodded. ". . . yeah."

"You know," I went on, "I did that once, too, right there in the hospital, with everyone cluck, cluck, clucking, and saying, 'unless you learn how to swallow, we can't take out this tube and give you real food.' And I didn't know anything more about how to swallow than I do about running."

"I guess you'll just wing it." Ted glanced at his watch. "What do you think of those?" He pointed at the shoes on my feet.

It was probably past closing time, or getting near it. A ray of light glistened on the gold wedding band he wore. No doubt he had kids at home waiting for him, along with supper too.

"You know," I said, "I never do things this way—try on something before I know the cost." I shook my head. "How serious are the damages for them?"

"Not too bad," he said. "That style's been discontinued, so

they're on sale, twenty-nine dollars. But how do they feel? Do they feel okay?"

"They feel great. It's like walking on air." I was already reaching into my fanny pack for my wallet and thinking again about where I could teach myself to run.

"North End Men's Softball," I read on the back of Ted's shirt as he turned to ring up the sale, taking both the shoes and my credit card. The softball reminding me of the granite wall along the ball field, down by the harbor. It was just at the end of the street. I could take the long way home, go by and check it out.

Now that I had the shoes, I had to use them, especially since now Ted would know if I chickened out. Not that he and I had ever talked before or were likely to again, but still, he would know.

JUST A COUPLE BLOCKS FROM THE WALL, I PASSED Green Cross Pharmacy. What if I stopped in and got an elasticized ankle support to wear when I ran. It wouldn't give me all that much structural support, but psychologically? I'd used one when I graduated myself from wearing the leg brace with its attached flexible-steel-shank shoe, so maybe running, too?

I stepped into the jam-packed store and was immediately greeted by a schoolkid who seemed to work there, materializing directly in front of me, and blocking my passage. "Can I help you?"

Upon hearing what I needed, he turned and scurried up a narrow aisle, leaving me to wait just inside the door. I looked around, amazed by how much stock filled the storefront.

"These?" He'd reappeared, holding out one each, small, medium, and large Futuro elasticized ankle supports

I glanced at the price sticker, thinking, Hmm, not bad. I chose the medium. "Perfect. I'll take this one."

He turned, the package raised high overhead leading me to the woman in back, behind the register.

What a production, I thought. But glancing at the merchandise we passed en route to the back of the store, I realized no customer could have found a thing unassisted. The tightly packed shelves crammed not so much with like commodities as with containers best fitting together to completely fill the space.

"A bag?" the woman asked as she laid my money in the cash register drawer.

"No thank you, I'll just add it to this." I pushed the ankle brace into the briefcase I still wore slung over my right shoulder, and then there was the plastic bag with my new running shoes, complete with the shoe box, all on my right side—my left hand lightly clenched, empty. I must look a sight, I thought, stepping out onto the sidewalk. Oh well, gotta have local color. I laughed to myself.

Just across Commercial Street were the wall and softball field. I looked at the wall, waiting to cross the street and it occurred to me just how very public learning to run between the softball field and Commercial Street would be.

Either the publicness would spur me on like a challenge, because so many besides Ted and me would know, or it would freeze me up with embarrassment over how ridiculous it must look. I latched onto "challenge," because if I allowed myself to think embarrassment, I'd never try.

As I got closer to the wall, I saw, even smoothed by time, wind, and weather, its granite surface—probably a Depression-era work project—was rough. I'd need to protect my hand somehow. I walked the length of the wall, home plate to mid-left field, mulling over how.

What if, I rested my right hand on the wall looking and thinking, I still had the leather mittens I'd worn skiing. Just wearing the right one would protect my hand. After a while, the stone would destroy it. But this was important, and maybe by then I wouldn't need the wall or the glove anymore.

What was the distance of the wall?—maybe a hundred, a hundred fifty feet? It wasn't far enough, but it would do to get started. Maybe once I could do this distance a bunch of times, I'd learn to run well enough there wouldn't be a "fear barrier" any more.

I walked the length of the wall, my right hand reaching out and brushing against the stone. That it was Wednesday— Hump day, I laughed to myself, downhill to the weekend— popped into my head. And Labor Day weekend at that. A three-day weekend would be perfect to kick off a running project like this. Three days of practice, without having to worry about work.

After Labor Day, I'd know how long it took—getting ready, walking to the wall, running, walking back, cleaning up, getting dressed—I'd have time to figure out how to fit teaching myself to run into my life.

Walking home, I thought about what I'd need to go running. I had the shoes—the box bumping against my right calf. I had plenty of socks. As the weather got colder, I'd buy a few pair of knee-high soccer socks to cover my shins. I still had my well-worn Wheaton shorts from college. For colder weather, I could pull out that pair of ratty-looking sweat pants I never wore and that gray sweatshirt. I had the leather mitten and my new ankle brace. . . What else could someone possibly need? I thought laughing to myself. Not much. The only thing left to do now was figure out how to do it. And figure out how to get my body to do it. The idea settled firmly at the pit of my stomach, heavy and resolute.

Six:
Day One

PEERING AT MY BEDSIDE CLOCK RADIO, I READ THE TIME: six-colon-zero-zero. Game time! Last night I'd set the alarm for seven, but it was Saturday morning, Labor Day weekend. I rolled to the side, reaching my legs toward the floor and thrust the covers off my shoulders, already sliding out of bed.

Just after I shoved my legs into my shorts and pulled on my T-shirt, my stomach rumbled. I always woke up hungry. Should one eat before running? Ten years was a long time to remember such details. . . Well, maybe a banana.

I finished chewing, swallowing it fast, hardly warming the kitchen chair before I moved into the living room, and lowered myself to the floor, my legs spread in a wide straddle, the sole of my left foot pressed flat against the baseboard.

Bracing it against the wall allowed me to get a full stretch on the long muscles in my left leg—heel through to my hip. Without the wall, my leg wanted to roll dink-toe, which only reinforced a synergy that inevitably led to twisting that ankle, something I definitely wanted to avoid this morning.

Leaning into the straddle, back straight, I pressed my nose toward the floor between my legs, pushing firmly and steadily, no bouncing, until releasing. Shifting the direction of the stretch, I leaned my chest and face along my right leg, my nose still an inch or so above that knee, eyes focused on the bend of my ankle. The goal was to press my right cheek and then my left against my right knee. Then I'd stretch along the left leg until I could press my right and left cheeks against that knee. Stretching was complete when I could touch first my nose and then one after the other my left and then my right cheek to the floor between my knees.

Even with some paralysis still, I was almost as limber as before, and more than most people. This morning, too, I ended by touching the tip of my nose, then brushing my cheeks against the floor between my knees. I was ready.

Before going to bed, I'd left my socks, shoes, ankle support, and an economy-sized jar of Vaseline in the living room on the wooden trunk I keep my shoes in and sit on to put them on. I remembered something about protecting my feet from blisters by slathering Vaseline on them. The last thing I needed was a blister I couldn't feel on my left foot, or one I would feel on my right. Trying not to overdo it, I coated my feet with Vaseline, pulled on my socks and the elastic brace over my left ankle, and worked my shoes onto my feet.

Standing up, I inhaled long and deep, doing my best to flush the jitters through my system as I reached for the fanny pack I had stuffed the night before with my mitten, some tissues, a dime just in case, and my house keys. What if I fell and hurt myself? Get going, I thought impatiently.

Once out on the sidewalk, I turned around to face the building and stepped onto the bottom stair of the front stoop. There was one more stretch yet—my Achilles. I rested my right hand on the handrail, only the ball of my left foot and toes on the stair tread, my heel hanging over the edge. My right leg I held extended, the toes loosely pointed. Relaxed, my right toes didn't touch, but would if tensed, in case my left foot slipped off the tread or the left leg reacted strangely, spasming, and got me into trouble.

Standing this way, my whole body weight pressed down through my left leg, stretching all the long muscles in the back of my leg. I alternated between a nearly straight and a more bent knee until the leg and foot felt stretched, holding each position for a "fifteen one-thousand" count.

My right leg, naturally comfortable, got the same stretch much faster. After finishing up with my right leg, I shifted back to the left leg, just to remind her. Stepping off the stoop, I began walking up Salem Street, toward the harbor, the white spire of the Old North Church brilliant against the September blue sky.

As I walked, I assessed my gait, "listening to" more than

feeling to how my left leg was doing. She seemed to be fairly loose, which was good, though I could hear the left foot striking the ground louder than my right, hear it slapping the pavement. My right foot landed almost silently, just as it was supposed to, stepping heel first through the foot and onto the toes. My left foot I could hear landing flat, like a solid block, no dorsiflexion in that foot, (no muscle synergy reaching the heel toward the ground, leading the foot through the step), slapping the cement sidewalk, despite years of working to regain a natural heel-toe step. If I concentrated only on walking, sometimes I could hear it in my bones, a stride, as the left heel reached for the pavement and touched before the rest of my foot.

Because I'd noticed my left foot slapping, I had to try to focus my attention and correct it. That was the way my rehab worked ever since I'd started making the rules. My rules were much stricter than any of the therapists'. I stopped walking and stood, rocking side to side, my feet shoulder width apart and my right hand resting on a signpost. This left-to-right weight shift reminded my body's neurology that ankles are gimbals allowing feet to remain firmly planted, even while my body above swayed off vertical.

I rocked side to side, then forward and back, then almost circular, pushing my body weight forward onto my toes, to the side, back onto my heels, and out to the other side, all reminding my legs and my feet what was possible. It wouldn't help me learn to run if I allowed sloppy walking. My steps could and should sound and feel more even, at least not "slappy." Sometimes, my gait came closer to normal and felt right. I called those times "moments of brilliance." Whenever such moments happened, I focused on them, concentrating on the sensations—inside and out. Sometimes passing by storefront windows I could see my reflection as I concentrated on the feelings, even the flavor of the moment trying to engrave the experience in my mind, to imprint each element in my body memory as well as in my intellectual memory.

Standing there on the sidewalk, hardly far enough from my apartment to say I'd begun my running project, I remembered my Feldenkrais instructor, Mia Segal, saying nine years ago, "Think like you're making a ballet foot."

When I'd frowned, not understanding the instruction. She explained, "think you are walking like a ballerina."

Imagine, she'd meant—but only imagine—walking with my toes turned out to the side. It was hard to do—exhausting for any period of time—but while I thought "ballet foot," though my feet didn't actually turn out, my left heel would seem encouraged to reach for the ground in advance of the ball of my foot and my toes. Thinking "ballet foot" seemed to trigger a dorsiflexion-like synergy, leading to a more normal gait. But it was like rubbing your belly and patting your head while chewing gum and blowing bubbles, impossible to keep up for long—especially when the rest of the world was active too: with other pedestrians around, cars driving the streets, people talking, doors opening and closing unexpectedly. . .

I stepped, right foot first, imagining it turned out to the side, intently "listening" as my right heel touched and I stepped through the foot; heel, through the arch, onto the ball and then toes, until I pushed off onto my left foot.

Now the left foot. Thinking Mia's "ballet foot," I concentrated on what happened. Did my left heel land on the ground before the ball, and then the toes? I "listened." While it wasn't perfectly symmetrical with the right, it did seem more even than before: now right again, then left—Pay attention, pay attention, I thought, focus, focus.

With everything else that needed attention—where I was going, watching for unevenness in the sidewalk, stepping over curbs and back up again onto the sidewalk, and noticing the scenery around concentrating so much attention on just moving forward was exhausting.

Early Saturday morning, the traffic on Commercial Street almost wasn't, I crossed with hardly a wait. Just the other side of the ball field, the harbor was almost flat calm, only the ripple of a breeze. And above me, the late-summer sky was clear—only a few fluffy fair-weather clouds, and the sun already lower in the sky—fall was coming—shone warm already but not hot.

Once across, I faced the beginning of my wall. Standing before it, my feet shoulder-width apart, I rocked gently side to side again while I took the mitten out of my fanny pack, working it onto my right hand.

I rested my mittened hand on the wall's edge, against the chiseled strip along the edge. My index finger could ride the strip, my thumb hanging over the edge, angling groundward.

I'd imagined striding off my unaffected right leg first, hoping that between the momentum of that first stride, my right hand pressed against the wall, and whatever effort came from my left leg, I'd manage to copy my right leg's stride and more or less follow with my left leg.

If so, if that worked—even sort of—I'd imagined I'd repeat it again and again, the length of the wall—each right leg "running" stride followed by some imitation by my left leg. With practice, I'd somehow teach the left leg to follow through, ever more like the right.

For a moment longer I stood beside the wall. With my right hand resting on it, left foot forward, I pushed my weight onto my left foot and back onto my right, then forward again, shifting my weight off my right toes onto my left heel and through my left foot, anticipating the weight shifts of running. Then again I rocked back, reversing the running stride. Going back and forth, like a rocking horse, I gave each rock forward a little more momentum.

I watched, looking down at the foot. Uh! As I pushed forward harder to where my left heel lifted off the ground, I watched as my ankle thrust out and over my little toe.

Not good. I'd have to watch that and rock the left foot forward to just before my heel left the ground which would be just before the ankle wanted to roll—more Feldenkrais strategy. With practice, I'd teach my left ankle to push through the left foot squarely, to push equally over the left big toe, balancing with the little toe without rolling that ankle. "If you know what you want to do, you can do what you want," the adage echoed in my mind.

And so, as I rocked again forward and back, just to that moment, I watched, listening to changes in muscles tension and in my body. I listened to what was involved in rocking: my right foot, ankle, calf, knee, thigh, hip, stomach, back, shoulders. . . everything.

And then, because it might be different, I shifted my stance to right leg forward, rocking front to back, hand always on the wall. I looked for the feeling in my left foot and leg, like what I'd felt in my right leg and foot just before it would be drawn forward into the next stride.

Returning to the left-foot-forward lunge, again and again I rocked. As the rocking and weight-shifting synergies began making more sense to the left side of my body, I pushed my hips harder, increasing the momentum, and more, until Now!

I thrust myself off my right foot, then fully onto and through my left foot, which forced me to bring the right leg forward in a next stride—then draw the left leg through. Now right, then left again, again . . .

A tiniest fragment of my brain recognized I was doing it! This concept of running was working!

Sort of, at least. My shoulders and upper body felt as though I was sitting a hard trot, everything jiggling with the stiffness of my gait. Somewhere deep inside, my mind focused on my left arch and ankle. Neither seemed to have the elasticity, the shock absorption, my right arch and ankle offered. Even my small bosom bounced uncomfortably. Oh well, I thought, laughing to myself at how foolish it was to notice that, and then laughing giddily because I was doing it! I was sort of running! After ten years of always bringing up the rear as everyone else hurried ahead of me, I was moving faster. And on my own steam.

"Okay, okay sweetie, that's a girl, good girl." I surprised myself, actually speaking the words out loud, coaching my left leg just as if she were separate from me—encouraging her to keep going—chanting in the steady one-two, one-two metronome beat my feet should have struck the ground with.

"You're doin' okay. Keep it goin'. Keep it going' Again, again. That's it. That's it. Good girl. More, more, come on . . ." I told my leg, coaching her, but not too loudly. I spoke deep and low, under my breath, the way I would have to soothe an infant or to urge a horse over a fence.

Hey, I thought, no one was there to hear me, why shouldn't I coach my leg? Measuring the tempo for the kids focused my attention, easing the tension.

And as my mind got involved with justifying encouraging myself out loud, Damn it! I caught the toe of my left shoe on the sidewalk, twisting my ankle, pitching me forward—doing just what I'd feared when I'd thought about teaching myself to run—falling. Oh ouch. Damn it

Damn. The moment I wasn't paying attention, look what happens. Ouch.

Resting my hand on the wall worked just as I'd imagined it would. Long before I came near crashing face-first onto the sidewalk, between my right hand, the wall, and my right leg I did it—I maintained my uprightness.

Looking back to where I'd begun, I wiped the pain-induced sweat off my forehead with the length of my forearm and swallowed hard. I wouldn't think about the twist. I'd gone only twenty-five, maybe thirty feet. But it was actually sort of running! No doubt it hadn't looked pretty, but what I did had been closer to running than walking! And it would get better.

I WAS READY TO TRY AGAIN, STANDING, MY LEFT FOOT ahead of the right. Once more I was rocking forward and back, gently, to start, my right hand palm-down on the wall. This time, I rocked knowing I could get to a point when momentum would thrust my right leg into a first stride, propelling my left leg to follow, and that if I tripped, I wouldn't get hurt. I'd catch myself with my right arm on the wall.

I concentrated on recognizing that moment just before my right foot left the ground, when my left leg received my full body weight, my right leg thrusting ahead and down until landing it pulled my left foot off the ground and through another stride.

I knew it would work. Impatiently, I ramped up the rocking, pushing harder, trying to move myself more quickly toward the thrust forward with enough momentum to get me going again. I had more wall ahead of me to get me farther.

"That's it, that's it," I told myself, my voice deep and

chanting again. "That's it. Okay sweetie," I told my left leg. "Come on, let's do it."

Forward again I rocked onto my left leg, as if I would follow with a stride from my right leg—one I could remember now, rather than just imagine.

Now! I recognized the moment this time and worked my right leg through the first stride, following with my left. Again—and, again—and, again—and . . . This time I tried standing taller, not rounding my back in a crouch so much, yet still leaning forward at the hip, my right elbow still flexed while somewhat straighter, ready again if needed. Maybe if I organized my upper body better I'd be less likely to trip.

Already I was playing with—well, experimenting with— how I carried myself, even while wholly focused on running.

"There, that's a girl, that's a girl, that's it, that's it," I said, my right leg pushing through, my weight momentarily supported on my left foot alone, though balanced with my right arm. "Come on, go on, girl, go on. That's it. That's it. That's good, good, good."

Right-to-left, left-to-right, right-to-left, though lopsidedly. It was a gait heavily supplemented by my right arm and the wall. And it probably wasn't technically running. But it sure wasn't walking, either. I knew what I did now was a lot closer to running.

"Forward, forward, keep on going. Forward, forward, forward," I chanted, my words a silent cadence in my head now. Keep it going, keep it going. Come on, come on.

And then there wasn't any more wall. Maybe it was fifty yards I'd just gone—not a huge distance, the length of the "dash" they made us run in grade school and junior high as part of earning the Presidential Physical Fitness Award.

It wasn't all that far, really, but my heart was pumping. I could feel the effort in my body—blood coursing throughout, muscles that hadn't been used that way in years, complaining. But I wasn't out of breath. At least I wasn't out of breath after only fifty or so yards of sort of running.

I turned around to walk back to where I'd started. Maybe when I got to the beginning of the wall, I'd try it again. Or maybe I'd go home and think about how I'd done what I'd done and about how to make it better.

Walking back, I noticed a slight strain in my abdominals. Almost instinctively, I rested my right hand against my stomach. I had remarkably strong stomach muscles, but still I felt their effort. I then reached around to my back, kneading the thick muscle beside my spine at my waist, my left latissimus dorsi. My lats and my abdominals seemed to have participated in my running effort most, even more than my leg muscles.

Hmm—interesting, I thought. Running on lats and abs. Better than running on empty, I laughed to myself. I knew this was going to be different—but running by my stomach and back muscles?

I'd walked back the length of the wall. Should I try it again? Already I could see more people up and about—driving past, walking dogs, even a couple throwing a Frisbee on the other side of the wall, in the outfield . . . What the hell. How would I learn if I didn't push? I was here, so go for it.

A single "run" of a few dozen yards couldn't be enough to exhaust me, could it? Certainly not. I turned around, repositioning my feet, hand on the wall again, and rocked back and forth, starting more vigorously, knowing better now how much momentum would push me forward onto a first stride. I was so focused, I didn't notice anyone.

"What are you doing?"

I looked, scanning to the side, trying to find the high young voice somewhere beside me on my left, in the nothingness of a peripheral blindness since the hemorrhage. Still rocking, I turned my head until I found him, a kid with a too big baseball mitt hiding one hand, the other pressed against his hip. I guessed he was probably six or seven years old.

Good for him, I thought—he had the confidence to ask. "I'm teaching myself to run," I said, as matter-of-factly as if I'd told him it was Swahili I was teaching myself.

He scowled. "Teaching?" he asked, parroting my verb choice. "Why don't you just do it?"

"I would, except for my leg," I patted my left thigh, "she doesn't remember how. She's partially paralyzed."

"Oh," he replied, still curious.

"Come on, Mikey, It's time to go. Don't you bother that lady," a woman's voice called out. I looked over to my right into the ball field and saw her just beyond home plate tethered to a dog, one hand on her hip, her feet still pointing toward the Waterfront condominiums.

"It's okay to ask, Mike. But I think you'd better get going with your Mom. Maybe when you catch up with her you can ask her about *paralyzed*."

He stayed a moment, studying me, digging his toe against the sidewalk. "Yeah, okay, maybe. Bye!"

Alone again, I returned to my rocking, forward and back, vaguely wondering whether those eyes were still watching. I pushed harder, until there was enough momentum, and the first stride, the next, and until . . .

"I think you're almost doing it!"

His voice came from farther away this time, closer to his mother, but not with her yet. I imagined him watching, his arms crossed at his chest, his curiosity overruling. And imagined Mom, who must be just about fit to be tied now. But I should be concentrating . . .

"Mikey. We've got to go. Come on now. Let's go. Now."

"Thanks, Mike," I called out. Okay, now you, I silently told my left leg, reminding her I was paying attention. Keep it going, keep it going. Just 'cause you have an audience . . . that's no excuse to get self-conscious, no excuse to screw up. Come on, keep it going, keep it going. Keep it going. Especially because you have an audience, keep it going . . . my thoughts reinforcing the one-two, one-two cadence my feet should have.

As Mikey and then his mom broke through my concentration and I imagined even just him watching, my left arm had tightened even more, frozen in a spastic right angle now, my fingers clenched in a hard little fist. Whenever I felt pressured to perform, it happened.

Usually when my arm reacted, I could just wrap my right hand around my wrist and forcibly straighten my left arm. Sometimes it would be so tight I'd even have to leverage the elbow on my right thigh. Forcing the arm straight and holding until the muscles stopped fighting would release the spasticity, easing the painful strain in my left shoulder. Now, with my right hand busy protecting me from a fall, I either had to stop "running" or figure out some other way. I hated to stop. I was only halfway along the wall, and though my gait was rough, was it really a tiny bit better already?

But my shoulder. It was so tight, it ached. Each step jounced making it worse. When it was this tight at home, I had to hook my left fingers around the chin-up bar in my bedroom doorway and hang, my body weight countering the spasticity.

If I wanted to keep going, I had to do something about my arm. What were my options? As the most sought-after babysitter in the neighborhood, I'd learned how effectively a deep, steady, even chant calmed babies and small children. Maybe arms?

"Settle down, girl, settle down," I intoned, focusing on my breathing. I inhaled through my nose Settle, holding the down, and exhaled girl through my mouth.

"Settle," Inhale. "down" hold, "girl," exhale. "Settle," Inhale. "down" hold, "girl," exhale. With each inhale, I imagined the bones pulling apart, lengthening, the same way my ribs fanned. On the hold, I imagined leaning on the pulling apart. On the exhale, I tried to imagine muscles throughout my shoulder releasing.

As I exhaled, I tried to visualize my left arm stretching long, down toward the pavement, feeling the lengthening all the way through the longest finger.

Even as I chanted low and deep, "Settle down, settle down girl," some other segment of my mind continued encouraging my legs: "Keep goin', sweet. Keep goin', babe. Keep goin', you're doin' fine. Keep goin', keep goin'."

Round after round of inhale, hold, exhale, and the pain in my shoulder eased some—though the muscles were still far too tense—but I was almost to the end of the wall.

Damn, damn, damn. Was it shifting attention to my arm, or noticing I was nearly to the end of the wall that had my left toe catching on the pavement and tripping me up again?

Stopped for the moment, I stood, left foot forward in the lunge again. Leveraging my left arm across my body against my thigh, I straightened it with my right hand then pulled it up and across, bringing my left fist even with my right shoulder. With the tension now released, I tried breathing the same release. Inhale, spreading the bones apart. Exhale, lengthening the muscles.

My shoulder managed, I rocked out the pain in my ankle

and, lunging forward, ran the last few steps. Once there, I began to turn around for the walk back to the beginning of the wall and then stopped, wondering What if?

My ongoing rehab, enhanced by Feldenkrais' theories sometimes involved reversing the sequence of what I wanted to do. What if I walked backward to the beginning of the wall? My right hand could rest on the wall, guiding and balancing me. Now wouldn't that "free my uprightness," as Feldenkrais practitioner Ruthy Alon would say?

If I could understand it—understand intellectually and physically and intrinsically, even emotionally, how to walk backward, at a deepest level I would understand walking, and I would know better what I wanted to do—running. Without a doubt, walking backward fifty yards on a public sidewalk would look weird, but how much weirder than what I'd already done? The point was to know what I wanted to do, so I could do what I wanted—to really know.

Walking backward along the wall after about ten years of focusing on just relearning to walk, and now run, felt Alice-in-Wonderlandy: unreal, confusing—Twilight Zoney—par for the course with the Feldenkrais Method.

I'd started stepping back right leg first, expecting it to know how, and concentrated on what happened. I concentrated on how my leg organized so the foot moved one pace behind me, on the sequencing of muscles involved. How did I lift my right leg? What happened in the hip, knee, quadriceps, hamstrings, calf, ankle, arch? What happened through the long foot bones attached to the toes, the metatarsals? And speaking of the toes, how did they behave? Oh, and what was going on in my torso—front, back, and sides?

When it was the left foot's turn, I heard the difference, the left toe dragging against the pavement. What was different? My right foot hadn't dragged. I focused, remembering, in my body memory, the synergies raising my right toes and simultaneously dropping my right heel (dorsiflexion) as the gluteal muscles in my butt drew my upper right leg back, all triggering an easy flex in my right knee. The left foot didn't raise high enough to clear the ground and step backward.

Hmm, interesting, I found myself thinking. So that's how it works . . . What a bizarre feeling—though familiar after so many Feldenkrais movement experiments, I thought, trying it again with my right leg, my left, and again, again . . .

My center of balance was off going backward. Bewildered, I moved more slowly concentrating on each step backwards until there was no more wall, and I was at the beginning again, ready to try running for the third time.

It wasn't such a long distance, but already, after just two goes at it, I noticed exertion in my quadriceps and, curiously, along the length of muscle in my back parallel to my spine, shoulder to hip—my left latissimus dorsi—and not so much the right lat, as well as in my stomach muscles. Had I used either my lats or abdominals to run before? Did able-bodied runners? I remembered only leg muscles, hips ankles, feet, buttocks, and lungs tiring from running.

Rocking forward and back, I edited the thought this

would be my last go at running for the day, to a *next run,* and rocked until Now! On the ski slopes, you only got hurt on a last run, so why jinx yourself with a "last run"?

Was there really a difference this time? I wondered as I "ran" beside the wall, this time silently encouraging my left leg. By thinking the encouragement, did it focus attention on my leg and help keep it going? Was my stride a tiny bit less jerky this time? And if it was, was the change due to walking backward, or was it practice—trying again and again?

At the end of the wall, I stepped into the center of the sidewalk, away from the wall, and began the walk home. Walking seemed so sedate, nowhere near the excitement of running, even the way I did it . . .

But as I walked, I could split my attention away from my forward movement and notice the leaves beginning to curl, rustling more noticeably in the soft breeze, a crisp undercut to the still warm temperature. Fall was nearly here, kids would be going back to school next week, summer was almost over. And I was teaching myself to run!

A ringing phone greeted me as I unlocked the door to my apartment.

"Hi, how'd it go?" David asked.

"I did it!"

"Good! maybe we'll go running together some time."

"Oh I'm nowhere near that yet. I've got a herky-jerky gait, and I very much need the wall to break the fear barrier."

"The what? You didn't fall, did you?"

I raised my eyebrows in response, even though he could-n't see me, and laughed. "Well, I tried to . . . "

"Tell me," there was an edge in his voice, so I laughed again. "Rolled my ankle some a couple times. It wasn't bad—the pain mellowed after the first jab, so I started again each time—like getting back onto the horse . . ." I left out reference to the sharp, stomach-clenching, "I-think-I'm-going-to-throw-up" pain that accompanied each twist, but he probably imagined it anyway, having seen my ankle turn before . . . "But I did three passes the length of the wall!"

"Umm, so how do you feel?" he asked. I noticed the lack of enthusiasm.

"My muscles are far too tired from just a short walk, sort of running a total of maybe a hundred fifty yards, and a short walk home. I must be in lousy shape."

"What muscles? Legs?"

"Believe it or not, not so much my legs as my stomach, back, and even my shoulders . . ."

"So what else is on for today?"

"I want to do some Haymarketing and maybe go to Open Studios over by South Station with Karan. How 'bout you? Are you up the hill in the office, working on such a beautiful day?"

"Yup. Maybe we can get together later, for dinner."

Seven:
Rules to Run by

IT DIDN'T TAKE LONG FOR ME TO SEE I NEEDED RULES TO make sure I kept this up—rules strong enough to make me get outside running, even when I didn't feel like it, rules that would get me out there in the rain, the cold, and heat—out there despite having twisted my ankle the last time out, and still vividly remembering it—rules that would get me out there despite a fall and maybe scraping myself on the wall. Now that the long weekend was over, I needed rules requiring me to get out running even on those days work didn't go well or when something else to do beckoned, rules that made me go running whether I'd gotten enough sleep the night before or not.

If I intended to teach myself to run well enough to

be able to run whenever and wherever I wanted—not always along a wall—I needed bona fide fire-and-brimstone rules. Otherwise, my running would end up just another cobblestone the road to Hell paved with good intentions. . .

So I came up with these three.

1) Tell everyone. Tell relatives—parents, grandparents, brothers, sister, in-laws, cousins, aunts, uncles, new friends, old friends, college friends, acquaintances, everyone. Tell them all "I'm teaching myself to run."

2) Wash your hair only after running, not even quickly touching it up in the sink—once I got to running far enough that I only ran every other day, if I just didn't feel like running, I'd have to go through the day knowing my hair should have been washed.

3) Running shoes may not come off your feet unless you've run. This wasn't quite such a public rule. No one but I would know if I broke it. But if it were a rule, it should help keep me from turning around and coming back without running, my mind changed just because of rain or cold or, in the winter, snow.

I THOUGHT MY RULES IN THE THIRD PERSON, in effect telling myself Thou shalt not, making them feel like commandments engraved in stone and handed down from a mount. The "shall/shall not" meant that while I was physically capable of not doing each, I didn't have permission.

Telling everyone meant that if everyone knew and asked about it all the time, I'd have to keep working at it and improve. Too many people would know if I gave up. And quitting publicly would be so much worse than just not accomplishing something only I knew about. If it turned out to be impossible, I'd get the "Atta Girl" for putting in the effort, but if I got tired of it and gave up prematurely, if I quit, everyone who meant anything to me would know. How would I live with that?

The hair-washing rule could be a very public consequence skipping a run. Once I got to running well enough and going far enough to need a full lay-day between runs, I'd only run every-other-day. With this rule, I'd just be allowed to wash my hair every-other-day. I'd long suspected daily hair washing was an advertising-based urban legend. But I also knew two days was the limit and that I'd have to get out there every other day. This rule also meant I might have to organize my social life around my running schedule. I could learn to say, "Gee, I'm sorry, Doug, tonight doesn't work for me," thinking I'd want to wash my hair before seeing you, and I can't do that until tomorrow after my run . . . . I could say, "How 'bout tomorrow night?" Nobody else needed to know about the second rule. But it had to be inviolable.

I thought not allowing myself to change my mind about running after the shoes were on my feet would help combat that last bit of inertia—the glance at the clock and thoughts about not going because it might take too long, because it was raining, or, as it got deeper into late fall and

55

winter, snowing, or because it seemed too cold. If I felt well enough, if I weren't too sick or too exhausted to roll out of bed and get dressed, then I was well enough to run. The rule was, once I got dressed and tied on my shoes, there was no turning back. Besides, I'd need to wash my hair . . .

After that first day, I no longer ate before running. Food sloshing around in my stomach felt awful. Besides, it seemed marathoners and probably most runners ate well the night before and then again after running. Once passing the get-up-and-get-dressed test on running mornings, I'd go straight to the shoebox, sit down and apply the Vaseline, pull the elastic brace over my left ankle, and tie on my shoes. Once I did all that, I had to go run.

The shoes rule also meant my running shoes weren't to be worn for anything but running. Designating them "running-only shoes" made them special, a part of the ritual that began with the alarm continued with the stretches, the Vaseline, the elastic support brace, leaving the apartment, and stretching my Achilles. Once started, my rules meant there was no turning back.

Eight:
Going Farther

Every day that week I'd run back and forth along the wall. Friday afternoon already and nearly sunset, and I'd just finished a fifth nonstop running of the wall, each time walking backward to the start. Though the toe of my left shoe still dragged, kkkrrhkkrh, across the sidewalk most times my left leg strode forward, just before my foot was supposed to flatten out parallel to the ground, it was time to find somewhere I could run a longer distance.

Exercise was supposed to happen only every other day, but I justified daily with the observation that a hundred-foot run followed by a hundred-foot walk backward repeated three and now five times couldn't possibly be strenuous enough to require full forty-eight hour layovers in between.

Twenty-four hours should be long enough to rest my muscles. Besides, daily practice seemed more important to kick-starting the learning to run than did rest. Once I progressed to running a mile, and then miles, I'd run every other day, allowing myself a full day between runs.

Just about every afternoon, one softball team or other had been playing in the field beside my wall. Sometimes I'd wonder whether I knew anyone watching or playing. It felt awkward, all those people potentially watching. What did it look like, a grown woman pushing herself to run back and forth, one hand on the wall? People I might know or who knew of me were bound to have noticed, and once they saw, did they wonder about my sanity?

It was past time to look for a new place to run. Somewhere with my still necessary handrail but where I could push myself a longer distance nonstop, somewhere I could build up my endurance with a distance long enough to work on my form.

At the end of my fifth fifty-yard "dash," instead of walking backward to the start before heading home, I continued past the end of the wall along the outfield and toward two sandy dirt strips cut into the grass well beyond left field. They looked about thirty feet long and four feet wide, bounded with railroad ties; the bocci courts.

No one was playing the traditional Italian sport that looked to me to have rules something like a cross between bowling and pool, played outdoors. I couldn't remember seeing these courts empty on a temperate, still-bright evening. Of course, for all I knew, the bocci season ended on Labor Day.

The gray-purple sand on both courts had been freshly swept and sprinkled with water—in anticipation of next season? or the next play? Older Italian North End men meticulously cared for and played on this small but heavily used section of Waterfront Park. I'd watched the game before but had yet to figure out the rules.

Just a little farther along, past the infield of a second baseball diamond, I turned right onto a path beside the Stirretti skating rink, heading now toward the harbor. Was this cement sidewalk path new? I looked down at the well-worn surface and decided no, just new to me.

As I got closer, hand on hip, I surveyed this portion of the HarborWalk. Along the harbor's edge walkway I found standard municipal steel-pipe railing—a perfect "fear barrier" breaker, except every five feet, the railing was interrupted by fist-sized vertical stumps, and along a section without stumps, the railing rose out of poured concrete footings which cut into the walkway two and a half feet, making it impossible to run close enough to hold the railing.

Behind the Stirretti Rink, the cement sidewalk merged into a well-maintained, weathered boardwalk—probably a far more forgiving footing than cement or asphalt. But for those vertical stumps in the railing, it was perfect back there—sheltered, private, with lovely vistas of the harbor. What could either those cement footings or the vertical stumps in the railing add to the structural integrity of the railing?

I gazed out over the harbor and for the first time noticed the all-wood, L-shaped pier, with its sturdy-looking though undoubtedly splintery wooden handrail. If I went out onto the pier, it would be at least four times the old distance. If I started running along the boardwalk, assuming I could learn to deal with the stumps in the railing, and then out around the pier, it'd be have to be maybe a thousand or more feet, nonstop. Eventually, I'd be able to go around again and again. The handrail lined both sides. I'd only have the width of the sidewalk to get across to make a second lap

And what a spectacular place to run: along the harbor, across from Old Ironsides tied up at a Charlestown Navy Yard wharf, and out over the harbor. Tomorrow I'd run this new route—maybe even twice. Even if it rained.

Nine:
The Causeway

I PICKED UP THE TELEPHONE RECEIVER HEARING ONLY the familiar background sounds of my parent's home. "Hi Mom," I said.

"How did you know it was me?"

I laughed. "Oh . . ." A week or so ago they'd gotten a cordless phone. Since then, whenever Mom called, she either hung up on me or waited silently a few moments before speaking, as if she didn't believe a disembodied handset could actually find me all those miles away in Boston. . .

"We haven't seen you in a while."

"Yeah, I know. I've been busy. Teaching myself to run, plus working full-time, all my regular rehab stuff, and trying to fit in a social life doesn't leave much time for visiting. I did buzz in and see Gram while you guys were up in Maine."

"Did you? When was that?"

"Umm, today's what, Friday? Not last Saturday, the one before. I was thinking about coming out soon. The running is still hard, but not as bad. I only run every other day, now that I'm going far enough to justify a day off to rest my muscles."

"How's that going?" Mom sounded cautious and not so enthusiastic. Couldn't blame her, though. She'd spent too many hours sitting vigil beside my hospital bed, waiting for the coma to let go of me, watched countless therapy sessions, and had listened over and over to my devastation about what used to be and no longer was.

"You're not going to hurt yourself, are you?"

"It's going great, and I even think I'm walking better, too. That's got to be because of the running."

She'd paused to take a breath, perhaps not even hearing me, before asking, "What are you wearing for shoes? Do you have good shoes?"

"I have a pair of running shoes and they fit beautifully. They're lightweight, give me great support, and I'm not allowed to wear them except to run." It was my turn to pause for a breath, but I quickly added, "One of my rules is, once I put them on, I can't take them off unless I've run."

"Does your doctor know you're doing this?"

"My internist does, and so does Marty."

"Okay kidduko, as long as you're not going to get yourself into any trouble."

"Who, me?" I laughed. "Trouble?"

"Yes, you." She knew me too well . . .

"Hey Mom, you know? I bet the breakwater along the Causeway would work for me. Tomorrow's Saturday, and it's a running day. I could hop on a bus and come down tonight or first thing tomorrow morning and do my running along the Causeway tomorrow morning."

"Tonight would be fine. I've got a beef stew cooking in the Crock Pot for supper, tomatoes, salad stuff, and zucchini from the garden."

"Better than I've got. By far," I laughed. "I'll pack my running stuff and be there in two, two and a half hours."

I hopped onto the rowing machine and then the leg weights, finishing up the daily rehab I couldn't do away from home. Everything else was floor exercises and stretching.

So, how does this work?" Mom had driven me to the Causeway, parking the car in the beach parking lot. We were walking together toward the start of the Causeway and the rough cement breakwater. I'd intended to walk there from the house, but that plan was swiftly vetoed—my sweats "weren't warm enough."

I'd thought I'd use the breakwater just as I'd used the wall along the softball field. I just hadn't remembered it as shoulder high, recalling it as about the same as "my" wall. And then there was the "pebbliness" of the cement they'd used to construct the breakwater. Would it ruin my mitten?

I shrugged, thinking, "oh well, we were there. I couldn't back out now, though the sharp autumn sea breeze, already whipping up whitecaps on the ocean side and raising Goosebumps on my arms and thighs, recommended turning back. We could just climb back into the car and return to the house . . . But I had my shoes on, and today was a running day. Besides, I wanted to wash my hair. I could always find another mitten—maybe try the left one on my right hand . . .

"Like this." I glanced at Mom. Her lips were pressed together in a not-at-all-enthusiastic firm line. I ignored her doubts. "I put on this mitten," I said, pulling it out of my fanny pack and working my right hand inside. My Achilles! I thought. Where can I stretch them? I panicked until I noticed the "No Parking" sign planted almost at the curb. "And then I stretch."

One by one I dangled my heels over the curb, my back to the roadway and my fingers wrapped around the signpost. "And stretch some more." I swept a shard of glass and some sand off the sidewalk with my right foot before setting down to sit on that sidewalk, legs straddled wide, my left foot braced against the base of the breakwater, hoping most of the stretch I'd already done before leaving the house was still with me.

"Then I rest my hand on the wall" I said, as I stood up.

64

Shoulder-high felt weird. It was a capped breakwater, with about eighteen inches hanging over the lower three and a half feet. I considered pressing my hand into the underside of the overhang, trying it as I arranged my feet, left foot a pace ahead of the right, but underneath felt even weirder.—so shoulder-high again. "Then I rock back and forth, like this," I said, demonstrating, "until I get the momentum to throw my right leg into the first stride."

Mom watched, standing near but not crowding, her hands pushed into the front pockets of her windbreaker. "But now that I've been doing this for a month or so, I usually don't need to rock as much as I did in the beginning. I think maybe because my leg is starting to figure out what she's supposed to do, and because usually I've gotten her started walking over to my running place."

I was starting to talk myself out of this. I'd been standing too long, even with rocking. Only the Achilles off the curb had felt like the stretches I did on my front stoop. I'd felt self-conscious sitting on the sidewalk, stretching, with Mom looking. Oh, shut up, I told myself, let's go.

"And harder and harder, like this, until my left leg figures it out and I can pull through the left foot as my right foot finishes its first stride." I demonstrated, striding again left, right, left, right, then rocking again.

"See you, Mom!" I called out, still looking straight ahead but knowing she watched though not knowing whether she shook her head or nodded, smiling. encouragement, the way she had when she'd witnessed my first few steps between par-

65

allel bars, my ankle and lower leg reinforced by an awkward leg brace, my feet clad in heavy leather orthopedic shoes, my right hand hanging onto only the right parallel bar.

"Oh, shit!"

Maybe I was embarrassed by the audience, maybe it was the higher wall, maybe a hole in the sidewalk, maybe I wasn't concentrating hard enough. Whatever it was, despite the elastic ankle brace, my left ankle rolled. Hard. Painfully.

A hard roll like that would happen sometimes just walking—even just in my apartment and often it did.

Each time it happened, it was a shock, and it hurt, a lot—a "gotcha-in-the-gut" hurt tightening up everything, a bending over at the waist hurt, a contracting left hip, knee, ankle, and arm hurt, a suck in a deep breath gasping hurt, a hugging arms together tight against my chest hurt. And a waiting hurt. Waiting for it to pass so I could start again.

"Oh, honey." Mom was hurrying behind me, having let me get a few paces ahead. "Maybe you shouldn't do this. You're going to hurt yourself."

I knew she'd never said anything like that when I was a little girl, first learning to walk and then to run. She'd let me fall, crashing to the ground, and then been there to pick up the pieces and wipe the scrape clean before sending me off again. Not that I'd fallen this time. I hadn't, just twisted my ankle. No blood, I thought. So no big deal.

I knew once I caught my breath, once I got past the pain, once I eased the tension shortening all the muscles on the left, somehow the ankle would be stronger—as if refocused. She'd be firmer, as if resolved not to let that happen again, at least as long as the pain was fresh in her ankle memory.

"No, come on Mom. Of course I'm going to do this. Look. It's a beautiful day—a bit brisk, but perfect for running. I've got the rest of the Causeway to do. I'm going to do the full half mile."

"And then what?" Mom looked doubtful.

"Oh ye of little faith!" I laughed. It was a favorite phrase of Dad's. "Then I walk back and decide whether or not to do it again!"

Ha! I thought. The length of the Causeway was probably farther than I'd tried yet. To think that I might do it again. Well, why not?

"Okay, enough gabbing. Dad would be telling us, 'when your mouth's working, nothing else is.'" I lay my hand on the wall, feet positioned again, and rocked. Atta girl, I thought, speaking to my left leg, Atta girl, rock. I thrust my weight through my hips, off my right foot and onto the left. Okay, baby, the words echoed in my mind. You can do this. Not a problem. Come on, girl. Feel the weight rolling through? Feel it press the heel into the ground, spring over the arch, onto the ball, onto the toes, and off.

I pushed with my right foot, bringing that leg through, until the foot was ready to receive my body weight, ready to take it through and then pass it to my left foot. Go.

Go on, go on. Yeah, yeah. Feels good, feels good.

67

Shoulders square, upper body centered. You can do this, I chanted silently, the steady beat for my feet to follow. My right foot struck the cement heel-first, then onto the ball until through the toes. Feel it? Feel it? I chanted. Copy, left foot. But still I heard the left foot slap the sidewalk, the whole foot together, not heel striking first. Come on baby, heel-toe. Heel-toe, I chanted silently, repeating remnants from Miss Bell's tap dance class decades ago. You can do this, I reprimanded myself. You can do this. You're going to do this.

I was nearing the end of the Causeway already. Apparently Mom had gone back and gotten the car. I was aware now of her flanking me, hugging the sidewalk, driving beside me. I'd sort of known she was there but hadn't had room in my head to think about it. Tune out the audience. Focus on one foot and then the other, I thought, remembering an old friend's, joking credo from so long ago—years before the stroke Forward, always forward—never straight.

At the end of the breakwater, I rocked back and forth a bit to ease my leg into finishing. It would have been better to walk back to the beginning, maybe even try it again. But Mom was there with the car, waiting. I got in.

Ten:

First thing in the morning

I NEEDED TO LEARN TO RUN. I SPENT MY WORKING DAY in a tiny cubicle studying a computer screen, talking on the telephone, and pushing through heaps of paper documents as a senior account specialist in the Problem Resolution Center of a major investment services company.

So far, I'd managed to fit in teaching myself to run after work. Typically, by the time I got home and changed, I'd step on the HarborWalk and then the pier in the middle of evening rush-hour smog and clamor. Some days, a cool, fresh sea breeze cooled from across the harbor. Other days, prevailing air currents wafted exhaust-laden air from stalled northbound traffic on the Charlestown Bridge over me. Already what was once new and interesting—the boardwalk and pier at water's edge—had become same old, same old and I needed a change. But what?

I thought I was getting better, but as with every aspect of my rehabilitation, improvement came in increments so minuscule I barely noticed. Day to day, I couldn't point to a single change. My left toe still kept scraping kkkrrhkkrh along the sidewalk with many of its strides. Yet when I looked at myself as if through someone else's eyes, compared with the first morning . . . clearly I'd improved.

Sure, I'd think, bored with the pace of rehabilitation, I was running better, but I still needed the handrail. After several weeks of this now same old, same old, I wanted variety. My route now consisted of two loops of the HarborWalk—I'd learned to lift my hand over the vertical stumps every five feet—out over the harbor onto the pier, around the pier, back to landside, along more HarborWalk toward the edge of the tennis courts, back to the start, and around again. Between walking down to my "running place," running my route, and walking home, I spent forty-five minutes to an hour.

I'd always been much more of a morning person than one with energy left over later in the afternoon. I was walking home from work on a non-running day thinking about how I could make it all work better. What if I shook things up by turning my schedule around? Maybe if I got up early and went out . . .

I had to be in my cubicle and logged in to the computer at 7:30 a.m., so I regularly got up at 6:30. If I planned to run before work, I calculated, I'd have to be stretched and out the door by . . . 5:15. Okay, so I'd get to see lots of sunrises coming up over the harbor . . .

If I'd spoken out loud to someone else, I'd have shrugged my shoulders, my lips pursed and head cocked to the side. I still needed to plan. To make this work, I'd have to get up at the same time every morning, so it would feel normal on running days. I'd run every other day and read, write, take care of my bills, straighten up the place, maybe even do my PT protocol on the mornings in between. I could think of any number of ways to spend an extra hour three or four times a week. Of course, sleeping would be an unacceptable choice, I thought, laughing to myself.

IT WAS A WHOLE DIFFERENT WORLD, THE VERY EARLY morning—five-fifteen, five-thirty a.m. A passenger car driving down Commercial Street was an anomaly, Traffic consisted of a taxi, a Globe or Herald newspaper truck, perhaps a bread or milk truck pulling up beside one of the neighborhood grocery stores, or a police car touring the area. That was it. I walked over to my "running place" refreshed, breathing deeply the cool, crisp, clean air.

The ambiance at five-thirty in the morning was better, but my route was way short. I still needed a handrail to run. The toe of my left shoe still scraped the ground, with many, though not all, strides. Running around and around in my odd loop, morning after morning, I was beginning to feel like a hamster on the exercise wheel in his cage. The sunrises were indeed spectacular, but I needed more nonstop distance.

Eleven:
Leverett Circle Overpass

"Good morning, Tommye Terrific. How's the running?" I picked up the phone to hear David ask.

It was about six a.m. on a not-running Saturday morning. I'd been up and dressed more than an hour, already a good way into my second cup of coffee, and writing. Sooner than I'd imagined, I'd finish writing one of my novels, then the next one and the next one and then there'd "just" be getting it published . . .

I laughed. "What are you doing up at this hour?" David's and my schedules were exactly opposite. He was typically awake throughout the dark hours tweaking a computer or pulling together yet another magnum opus brief and switching off lights and powering down equipment just as I was waking up to my alarm.

"I thought maybe you might want to get together for breakfast this morning."

"You're in luck, you know. I actually haven't eaten yet—just coffee." I waited a moment for his ever-ready response. "Yuck, coffee."

I glanced at the words on the screen in front of me. No, that doesn't read right, I thought, reaching for the mouse, but then David asked, "The IHOP? How 'bout I pick you up in about ten minutes?"

"You're on." My attention ripped away from the words on the computer screen and back the phone call. "I'll start timing you when we hang up," I laughed. David was always late, though if you asked, he'd insist he wasn't. "Catch you in a few. I'll be sitting on the front stoop, waiting."

Part of me hated to stop writing. There had to be a way to fit everything in: writing, running, friends, spontaneity, fun—oh, and a full-time job. Clicking the mouse, I set the cursor on that place, reworking the words that had bothered me, and then I returned to the end of the line. I still had a few minutes before I had to shut down the machine.

*

"FANCY MEETING YOU HERE," I SAID AS I STEPPED OFF the curb and pulled open the car door.

"Was I about ten minutes?" We were already moving toward the North End's main drag, Hanover Street.

"Close . . . depending on whether it was ten minutes driving or ten minutes from when you hung up the phone." I chuckled. "But not to worry. I used the differential well."

Turning off Hanover onto Cross Street, the first decision had to be made fairly quickly. "Na-no," I said, "don't turn onto Blackstone Street." On any other day, getting up and over the city streets would be the best way to get out of town. "It's Saturday, the pushcarts are out there."

"Right." David steered the car past the first turnoff, going out and around to get up and over on the elevated Artery.

I settled into the passenger seat, watching the road, enjoying the ride. Always I tried to understand what would come next, trying to connect where we were with what had come before and to anticipate what would come next. Since the hemorrhage, I no longer had the ability to automatically orient myself geographically, a function the neurologists called "spatial orientation." So, post-hemorrhage, I was often lost, when once my sense of direction had been a given.

I studied the facade of the old Boston Garden as we drove past, and just ahead the grassy knoll with the billboard sign promising "Affordable Housing Coming Soon." Catching a glimpse of a Storrow Drive sign a bit to the left, I thought David might take that route. Instead, he stayed right.

"While we're over here, I just want to take a look at something. A little farther up, on the Cambridge side, they're putting up some luxury condos where the rail sidings and stuff used to be. I want to see what it looks like."

I hadn't heard about this project, but it was Cambridge. Keeping up with what was being built in Boston was enough of a challenge. I glanced at the street sign for the right we took instead: Lomansey Way. Shrouded by the elevated Green Line T (Boston's rapid transit system), it was a dark, congested, six-lane roadway, interrupted intermittently by the legs supporting the tracks overhead. Typically, I crossed only the end of Lomansey Way on my infrequent trips to the supermarket. Driving down, I realized I didn't know what was on this street.

I watched carefully, curious to see what we'd find on the other side of Lomansey St. There didn't seem to be anywhere I'd want to go: a parking garage, more construction over behind the Garden. Until, "look—look at that!" I exclaimed, completely turned in my seat.

David slowed the car, glancing at where I pointed. There was almost no one else on the road, and it was a wide street.

"What are you looking at?" he asked.

"That pedestrian ramp! It's perfect!" I traced the long footbridge's gentle grade up and over a complicated intersection connecting to a T station before traversing several streets and tending back down to street level with my index finger. It seemed to go on forever and with handrails on both sides. "Look at how far it goes."

"What would you use it for?"

"Running," I said my eyes not leaving my discovery.

"It's a much longer walk over here . . . "

"It didn't take us much time to get here, and just look how far I could go without having to stop, and there's even those few stairs, off to the side at the bottom, I can use to stretch before and after."

Clearly amused at my excitement over such an ordinary urban structure, David glanced at the pedestrian overpass. He still didn't seem to understand why, if I could walk okay and as far as I wanted, running was such a big deal.

I kept my eyes glued on the overpass still longer, wondering which T station it was. Undoubtedly I'd been through it as a passenger on a train—I'd probably been to most of the stations on the system, at least stopping with the train if not getting out. I just couldn't remember ever walking across that overpass and boarding or leaving a train there.

"Shall we go?"

"Um, yeah." As we moved back out into the street, continuing toward Cambridge, I was able to read T signs for *"Science Park"* station. Then we drove past the Science Museum, and I realized that for four years I'd lived just fifteen minutes away.

"So when do you think you going to try running on the Leverett Circle Overpass?" David asked.

"Is that what it's called?" What a surprise. After years and years of subjection traffic reports lamenting tie-ups at Leverett Circle, and I'd never known it was just over here. "Tomorrow morning."

I WAS OUT THE DOOR AT FIVE-TEN. IT WAS SUPPOSED to have been five-o'clock, because I didn't really know how long it would take to walk to my new running place—but schedule slippage . . . It had taken longer to stretch my muscles this morning. Nervousness about going somewhere new? Who could tell with stroke-paralyzed two-year-olds?

A little extra tone this morning? I'd observed. Okay kids, now we're walking over to the Science Museum for a nice long run.

This early, the only activity was in the bakery next door, where they'd been baking all night and it was time to deliver hundreds of bread loaves all over the city. Crossing away from Prince Street it occurred to me I'd never noticed how much wider and in better condition the sidewalks were in this side of the neighborhood.

A police cruiser and then another drove past as I walked along the dingy North Station and Boston Garden–area streets. Five-fifteen was too early for the unsavory characters who frequented this part of town later in the day and at night. The cruisers and thoughts about the people who usually frequented this part of town made me conscious of my ratty, pre-hemorrhage gray hooded sweatshirt and many-wash-faded, once green, hand-me-down sweatpants. Probably, I thought, I looked as bad as the homeless people I passed sleeping on grates and I did sort of stagger.

It occurred to me how bad that was. Maybe those cruisers weren't just on regular patrol. If I planned to come this way regularly, I'd have to clean up my act and wear something decent. I'd need something bright early morning drivers would see and the cops would come to recognize.

But for this first day, I looked the way I looked, so I picked up my pace, walking even more purposefully down Causeway Street to Lomansey Way and my pedestrian overpass.

IT WAS PERFECT. I PAUSED AT THE FOOT OF THE THREE steps to the pedestrian walkway leading up and over the mess of intersecting roads and read the highway signs, familiarizing myself with the place: "Storrow Drive," "Charles Street," "Lomansey Way " and "I-93 to Logan Airport." At this hour, the roads were quiet. I slid my right hand into the mitten and studied the walkway. The handrails were perfect—waist-high smooth steel pipe on both sides, no more running only to walk backward to the start to do it again. The gradual turns the walkway snaked to make the slope curved gently. Someday I'd learn to take those turns at a run.

Already I was rocking forward and back, my feet a stride apart, right foot in back, my hand on the rail beside me. As I rocked, building up the momentum, my eyes traced the route ahead. I'd go straight, round the first curve, straight again, around another curve, straight again, then follow the pathway left, which would bring me opposite the "T" station around another curve and down the spur to the station.

Just before entering the station, which I didn't want to do (I was going for a run, not a ride . . .) I'd step across the walkway and run backtracking out to the overpass and run the long part toward the state police station and down to the sidewalk out onto to the Esplanade, beside the Charles River.

Running the first leg and spur until I was facing the station went just as I'd imagined, I crossed three steps to the railing on the other side, ready to get going again. Crossing the width would be where I'd begin teaching myself to run without the railing, I thought. Already I was going farther without stopping, my right hand sliding along a smooth railing—no stumps! It felt great. With more distance, I could play around and adjust what I did. I had time to think and to try reaching out with a longer stride, maybe encouraging my foot to land heel first, time to check that my vertebrae stacked vertically one atop the other, centering my upper body—left to right— and to adjust when they weren't. More distance even allowed me to try shifting the alignment of my head, and to explore what happened when my chin tucked in and to explore what happened to my gait when I jutted it out some.

Once across the walkway, I laid my right hand on the railing. All over my body I could feel the effort differently—in my calves, quads, and hamstrings, in my stomach muscles, and in my left latissimus dorsi.

Okay, I thought, enough standing around noticing differences. Rocking back and forth only a bit, I started off again. I must be getting better at this—building momentum to get going wasn't as important anymore. I ran beside the railing, my right hand riding along it, part of my mind still focused on the running I'd just completed. Was it a longer nonstop distance? Or maybe my muscles noticed the gradual slope riding up and over the traffic circle. My route over by the harbor had been level terrain

Before the hemorrhage, had I ever thought about how my legs, ankles, and feet handled changes in grade? Oh sure, I remembered working harder, my muscles complaining more, and even sweating more, but had I thought about better organizing my body to handle grade? No. It must have been reflexive then, an adjustment my body made naturally, without conscious consideration.

But now, as I started on the flat over the Leverett Circle intersection, still a ways to go before the walkway sloped down to the street, I began focusing on my feet. What had it felt like a few minutes ago, when I ran as the walkway rose gently upward? If I could re-feel how it was maybe I could imagine how it would be when the footing sloped down, maybe . . . I "listened," feeling more than hearing, how my right foot struck the ground with each step. I concentrated on how the heel struck first, on the "give" in my ankle and knee, on the push through the long bones of my foot, the metatarsals, and on rolling through my foot onto my toes, propelling me forward onto my left foot.

As my left foot stepped onto the walkway, I studied what happened, comparing it with my right foot, conscious of how very far from even, left to right, my gait was. Stride after stride, I concentrated my attention on the how and why.

What was the difference between the way my legs and feet responded to this running idea? Was it primarily my compromised proprioception (my awareness of where my leg was in space), the transient numbness throughout my left leg and foot, masking my perception of my left side? Of course, the difference would be due in large part to residual spastic muscle tone throughout all my joints—hip, knee, ankle, and throughout my foot, no matter how much stretching I did.

Seeing what I looked like running would probably have helped me understand what I needed to adjust, but since there wasn't a camera crew kicking around, I'd have to figure it out based on what I could see, what I heard, and what I felt.

But it was working. I was figuring it out. Each time I practiced, a tiny bit more bout running seemed to make sense. I looked up, breaking my focus on my feet, aware now of where I was and realizing the "downhill" had just happened. I'd been so concentrated each step, so focused on understanding how my right foot did it and on trying to make my left foot copy. Already I was approaching the entrance to the T station again. There was still distance left to run before I got back to the start. It was hard not to get lost in concentration here. The handrail was smooth all the way—no more contending with those stumps every five feet or so, as in the section of railing along the HarborWalk; no splinters, as in the railing around the pier; no roughness, as in the granite wall surface. The footing on the cement pedestrian overpass surface wasn't as forgiving as the boardwalk and the wooden pier, but it was well maintained and gently graded.

Eventually, with practice, I'd be running round and round my new track, building my endurance to miles. First, though, I had to finish this lap, and maybe I'd go around again.

Oh, damn! Ouch!

Yes, I was holding on, but this time my whole left leg got involved in the twist, beginning with the big-toe side of my shoe, rolling around onto my little toe. It hadn't quite cleared the pavement, pivoted, and forced my ankle to roll out into the handrail, taking my knee with it.

Hanging onto the handrail, I'd tried to control the fall. But thwack! My head cracked against the railing, catching the top of my ear and my right temple. Damn! my ear! my ankle. My whole leg—hip, quads, hamstrings, knee, calf—was in complete contraction. I hung onto the handrail, my body suspended over the walkway between my right arm and leg.

Damn, that hurt—all of it—my head, my ear, my ankle, my knee, even my left arm and shoulder were contracted in sympathy with my left leg. If I could just ease myself down to sitting, if I could sit there and straighten my left leg along the ground, if I could lean over to massage the ankle and then stretch again to get my leg psyched up and okay to try running again . . . Oh, and if I could rub my temple. Hopefully my hair would cover any lump or bruising I thought as I wondered, was my ear bleeding?

I'd chosen an even more public place to learn to run—commuters to Mass. General and Spaulding Hospitals and the Mass Eye and Ear got off and on the train here. Though it wasn't yet five-thirty in the morning, I saw two women approaching from opposite directions, two women who probably wouldn't have spoken more than a quick "Good morning" to one another when passing, who'd witnessed my crash.

They'd never leave me sitting there. I'd fallen in public enough times to know anyone who saw always wanted me back on my feet before they continued on their way. And they always yanked on my left arm to help me up—painfully unhelpful help.

"Oh, oh," the first one to reach me said. Not far behind I could hear the other coming, her polished nylon coat rustling like the petticoats Rhett had bought Mammy. "I saw the whole thing," the first woman said, reaching out to me. "What happened?"

I looked up at her, making myself smile. "I fell." It's not like this was the first time I'd fallen, I thought, saying nothing, focusing instead on where and how I hurt. I just needed to stay still a moment and settle down "the kids."

"Well, here, let me help you get up." She grabbed my left arm just above my elbow, pulling up and out as if it were a chicken wing she was trying to rip away from the carcass.

"Na-no. Please, please don't."

Between the tone in my shoulder and the angle she'd chosen to pull, it hurt—a lot. Tears glistened in my eyes from this new pain in my shoulder. She stopped but still held my arm in the same "tear the chicken wing off" position, leaving me with "stretched muscle too far/strained ligament pain," I'd deal have to deal with. Why didn't people ask what they could do to help instead of assuming they knew?

I didn't want to get up just yet, but it would be the only way to move these ladies on—I could hear the second woman fast approaching as I drew my right foot in under my hips, a bit left of center, scraping the edge of the sole on the pavement. I'd landed in an awkward position. Grown-ups didn't get themselves tangled up like this. But between my right arm on the railing and my right leg, I could haul myself to standing and ease the first woman's kind intentions. Once I was on my feet, she'd let go of my arm, since such intimate contact with an upright stranger wasn't polite.

"Did you break anything?" The second woman was finally standing over me, crowding around the way people do whenever there's a person down, but also, thankfully, blocking the sun.

God, this is embarrassing. How come the Wicked Witch of the West had a trap door when she needed it, when disappearing was the only graceful exit? "No, no," I assured her, smiling, "nothing's broken., I'm fine—really." I made myself laugh. "Just a little startled, that's all."

They stood there, staring at me, waiting. Clearly, neither intended to leave before I was standing, until I'd proven nothing was broken.

Okay, I thought. Upsy-daisy. I rolled my hips over my right foot, pressing my weight into it, and pulled up with my right arm, rising to standing.

"Thank you so much for your concern," I told them, "but I'm fine—really." I continued smiling, because it seemed important to reassure them. There was nothing they could do now. I'd fallen, but I was upright again. "It's a bit of a jolt, falling like that. Thank you so much for stopping. I really do appreciate your concern."

Slowly they turned, two strangers walking to the subway entrance together, heads already tilted toward each other. I heard them speaking animatedly—perhaps about me, though they could have discovered something in common.

Undoubtedly, after passing through the turnstiles, upon reaching the platform, one or both would turn around to check on me. For some reason, I felt a responsibility to do something to prove to them I truly was all right before they stepped onto the next train.

Man, my shoulder really bothered me—between the sympathetic spastic tone from the fall and that foolish woman yanking on it. If I started stretching out the tone, stretching the shoulder the right way—as opposed to the ripping it out

of the socket way—it would feel better. . . I lay my left hand
on the railing, arranging my left fingers, with my right hand,
so they clasped the railing and shifted my feet in line with my
shoulders. Then resting my right hand on top of my left, holding the fingers on the railing,. I then leaned my body weight
away from the railing, pulling on my shoulders.

Stretching out the tone this way would relax the fingers on
my left hand, and as they became flaccid, they'd slide off the
railing unless I held my them in place with my right hand. If
I had a good stretch going—if I really hiked out, so the pull
went all the way through my left arm, through my shoulders
and back, down to my pelvis—loosing my left hand's grip on
the railing could send me right back down, butt to the pavement again.

With all this attention to my left hand, my leg was settling
down on her own. She stood comfortably, supporting her full
share of my weight.

Both shoulders lightly rounded and relaxed, my head
tipped forward, eyes on the ground between my feet, I
stretched my arms, pulling away from the railing, my upper
body weight gently and constantly stretching muscles all the
way from the waist up. I stood holding, holding, until, at the
apex of the stretch, I gently shifted the pull to the right, holding, holding, until shifting to the center again and holding,
holding, then shifting left. I stretched through the full range of
shoulder movement, easing the tone in my back too, the tone
in my left lat.

WE-ELL, THIS FIRST TRY AT THE NEW PLACE WASN'T GOING as smoothly as it maybe could have . . . But at least here, there was still distance to run before I got down to street level, where I started, and where I could decide whether to head back home.

I glanced at my watch, five-fifty. Enough standing around—it was past time to get going. I rocked back and forth again until I was off again—not quite Derby speed, but there you go, there you go, nice, nice, nice, I told myself. I focused attention on my footsteps, thinking also about moving myself along a bit faster. Hmm, my left toe didn't seem to be brushing the walkway surface as much. Could it be I was picking up my leg better? Maybe twisting my ankle had taught her a lesson—for the moment, anyway? Good girl, good girl. Keep going. Good girl.

So what was it that was different this time? If I had my other hand, the left one, or if I didn't have to hold onto the railing, I could hold my hand over my left lats just to know what was happening. If I didn't need the railing, I could rest the palm of my right hand against my stomach and feel what was happening there, feel how I used my abdominals. In freshman choir, Chas, the director, had showed us how to feel our voices supported by our stomach muscles by resting our hands over our stomachs and to feel the difference between supporting and not. Regrettably, my one hand was already occupied by holding the railing, just in case . . .

Keep it goin', keep it goin', I told myself. I was already turning the corner and entering the slope downward to street level. Now that I'd noticed the slope, it was better, having thought about it in advance—or was slope just not a problem? Evie, our horseback-riding instructor, made us ride downhill sitting back in the saddle. She said it helped the horse balance better. Was I leveraging my upper body back ever so slightly? Did it somehow encourage my foot to touch down heel first and not catch my toe?

Some body leveraging to help with proper sequencing might be okay, but ever so subtly. Or maybe not at all. Maybe, as with Mia's ballet foot, simply thinking "sitting back" was enough to make it happen, enough to encourage my left foot to land heel first.

Somewhere I'd read that running in too upright a posture strained Anterior Cruciate Ligament in the knee. Actually leaning back even slightly would be like standing more than upright. I already knew about ACLs having torn my left one skiing. But that was another story, I reprimanded myself. I had to stay focused.

Where should my behind be? I remembered all those runners I'd watched, and thought about how runners crouched, some more than others. How much was correct?

I tried thinking back. What had I done before I got two kids permanently attached to my body? I couldn't remember. Ten years was a long time.

The handrail ended as the pedestrian overpass emptied onto the sidewalk. I glanced at my watch. No time for dawdling here, and I definitely needed a shower. Breakfast, too. I'd worked up an appetite and a sweat.

My new route was excellent. I could keep running long enough to really examinc what I was doing, to consider how my left side felt in comparison to my right, and to make adjustments. When things felt better, the overpass was enough nonstop distance to focus and really understand what might be different, long enough to lock sensations of "better" in my body memory, so perhaps I could call up "better" next time and do it. That would be key, engraving in my memory how it felt when my movement was "better" than it had been.

"Better"—but certainly not perfect. I had a long way to go before perfection. My left leg still didn't bend as close at the hip, and I couldn't raise my left leg as high as the right. Maybe my hip even swung my leg out to the side with each stride, though I wasn't conscious of it. I could feel my left knee didn't cycle through reaching my foot as far forward and taking as long a stride as the right. The sound of my footsteps wasn't an audio replay, one of the other.

But it was better. Definitely better. I attended to how the running felt, how it sounded to my ears and inside me, how it tasted inside my mouth, and how it smelled in the air around me. There was no salt in the air. It smelled like fall and winter coming soon, and like fresh water—the Charles River behind me now.

Twelve:
Filene's

BRIGHT WINTER SUN SHOWERED THE STARK ASPHALT circular driveway in front of the World Trade Center. But it did nothing to warm the wind whipping bright plastic banners trying to make the austere cement building a bit more festive. I stood alone, rocking side to side the way I always did, my toes pressed over the sidewalk's curb seam, waiting for the State Street shuttle van that was supposed to leave from here every fifteen minutes, and contemplating the impossible chore I hoped to accomplish. By now, my hour for lunch left me, at best, fifteen minutes to rifle through clothing racks, trying to find the suit I'd look reputable running in. If only Ted had what I needed at Sports Magic.

I could never imagine stranding hundreds of employees—

a couple thousand, perhaps—in an isolated warehouse building across Fort Point Channel a mile or two away from civi-
lization as we know it. Oh sure, Jimmy's Harborside restaurant was next door, there was a Shawmut Bank down the
road, and Anthony's Pier 4 restaurant. But no street life, no
drugstore, no place to get a haircut, take dry cleaning, buy
shoes, gifts, or running clothes—the errands lunch hours are
supposed to be used for.

If I were lucky, the van wouldn't take forever to arrive, it
would be a fast trip downtown, a quick walk up Washington
Street, to Filene's—not the basement, but the department
store. God knew where inside—Filenes's was five or six
floors of merchandise. I'd have to find a sales clerk in per-
fumes near the door to direct me.

"Yes, fourth floor." The tiny, tightly coiffured woman
pointed in the general direction of a space between clothes
racks that dead-ended at a floor display. I cut around trying
to follow the direction her finger had pointed toward access
to the fourth floor. No such luck. I got lost in a confusing
array of mirrors, racks, and men's clothing, and accessories—
not an "elevator" sign anywhere.

"And the elevator is . . . where?"

"It's right over there. Straight in front of you on the other
side of the men's department." From the tone of her voice,
obviously I was supposed to just know.

Damn it, they couldn't have made this more difficult,
could they? "Straight in front of you" was a Plexiglas men's

necktie rack—if it hadn't had all the neckties hanging on it, maybe I could have seen where "straight in front of you" would be. With fifteen or twenty minutes to find and buy a running suit and a few minutes to get to the van and back to the World Trade, I followed a serpentine route as "straight in front of you" as I could. Once I got through the men's department, I found it, reading the tastefully lettered word in two-inch red characters printed on the white wall:

ELEVATOR.

Stepping off the elevator I stood a moment surveying what I could see of the fourth floor. Hmm. Whatever department I needed wasn't immediately apparent. The electronic sounds of a cash registered caught my attention. I walked over to the cashier just as she finished ringing up and bagging a sale.

"Oh yeah, right over here." She said, leading me to the rack. "We don't have much left—it's last season's, but what's here is marked down, thirty percent off."

"It's an awesome thing," I said, laughing a little, "when exactly what I need is also on sale."

I surveyed the rack. Yes this was what I had in mind—bright "joy of exercise" neon colors. Reaching into the rack just past my size, I pulled out one of the suits. The idea was to get the brightest and, yes, most fun-looking nylon outfit, with a polyester/cotton lining. The hot pink one with black and lime green panels at the raglan-sleeve shoulders fit the bill best. I draped the suit over the rack, catching the hanger so the suit hung out over the others on the rack and started the zipper. I'd long ago learned the only way to deal with a jacket zipper one-handedly was to zip it an inch or so and pull the jacket over my head. Since I planned to wear this jacket at least three times a week, if I couldn't easily pull the jacket on over my head, it wasn't the one for me.

"Here, let me help you," the sales clerk offered as she reached up and began pulling the back of the jacket over my shoulders.

"No," I said, firmly but politely, speaking to her from the awkward position of the jacket neither on nor off my body but rather somewhere in the middle. "Thank you," I continued, "but if I can't get into this jacket by myself, then I'll not be able to wear it. You won't always be available to help me dress."

Peering out from under the jacket I saw her nod, her eyes opened wide.

I struggled with the partly-on jacket—I'd had to stop her helping me at the worst possible stage. As I wriggled, freeing myself of the jacket I heard her say, "I'm sorry."

"It's okay," I replied through the hot pink nylon. "How would you know if I didn't tell you?" Educating people always seemed to happen at the most inconvenient times.

I started again, laying the jacket over the rack back side up, inserting my paralyzed left hand and arm through the waist opening, threading the hand toward, into, and through the sleeve, my right hand guiding the process. Once the fingers of my left hand poked through the elastic cuff, I slid my right arm into its sleeve and then ducked my head inside. So far, so good . . . As long as my shoulders slipped fairly easily through the elasticized waist, this one would be a go.

Not a problem—the thing slid right over. A few tugs in the back and front, and the shoulders settled over mine—perfect. Now if only the pants fit too.

A quick minute in the dressing room—I pulled the elastic waist pants on over my pantyhose, just lifting up the skirt to look—and I was calling the cashier over to the register, my credit card already in hand—I was just about out of there. The price was as right as it probably could be without my having spent time shopping around.

MISSION ACCOMPLISHED WITH FIVE MINUTES TO SPARE . I walked around my supervisor's desk carrying my new nunning suit. I'd try it out tomorrow. No way the North Station–area cops could mistake me for a vagrant wearing this outfit, I thought as I rounded the corner to my cubicle. Hey, a girl has to worry about these things. If anything unsavory should happen during an early morning run, I sure wanted Mr. or Ms. police officer to know which side of the law I was on. . .

Thirteen:
Thanksgiving Morning

FILLED WITH FAMILY, FRIENDS, AND NEARLY ENDLESS COURSES of food, none prepared by me, and a running day to boot—this Thanksgiving had all the ingredients of an excellent holiday. And to cap it off, I intended to stretch my distance another lap. Thanksgiving had come at the perfect time. On a holiday or weekend day, I could add annother lap without worrying about being late for work. With a Thursday holiday, I could do the extra lap again on Saturday—maybe even Sunday too. By then, I could really get the new timing down.

We were expected at my folks' about noon for the cocktail party get-together following the traditional high-school football game. It was the annual gathering of extended family and close friends, followed by Thanksgiving dinner. Between the half-mile walk to the house from the bus stop, my run and adding another lap—I looked forward to being able to eat anything I wanted, without consequences.

The alarm went off at the regular time and, as usual, it was still dark. Why not relax a few minutes and go out a little later this morning? Surely I shouldn't be yawning in my aunts', uncles', cousins', and grandmother's faces. They were uncertain enough about my running. Hadn't I nearly died from a cerebral hemorrhage? Was running a good idea? Was it good for me? Was it safe? they wondered.

Since I'd begun running mornings and been up and out at the crack of dawn, right after the alarm woke me already a couple months now, so lounging in bed a couple extra hours, felt odd. At the princely hour of six a.m., I'd throw off the covers lest I be caught getting soft . . .

Even as I lay awake listening to a BBC report on the radio, I still trained, thinking about running. Lying there I imagined the sounds of running—my footsteps, the chafing of my nylon pant legs, the nylon sleeves under my arms, the hem of the jacket rubbing against my pants, my hair brushing against the collar, and the sound of my breathing, no matter how hard I tried to control it. Remembering breathing led to thinking about the kinesthetics of running, the feelings throughout my body, the muscles inside, and the bones, and the feelings on my skin. I thought about how it was now and imagined how it should be, based on how I remembered it being and on what I had seen in other runners.

Particularly the feet. I lay back, now thinking of running feet, even though I'd never been at all enamored of feet, having always thought they were rather funny looking. While feet may not be where running begins, I mused, they're close to the beginning and are intricately involved all the way. In my imagination, I sequentially examined how my ankle needed to flex to reach the heel to the ground and then extend to push the toes away (plantar flexion into dorsiflexion). From the ankle, my mental picture moved into how the length of my feet, the metatarsals, followed the leverage from my heel through my arch onto the ball of my foot, until my toes pushed off, powering the next stride, I pictured how it should look, imagining and feeling the stability throughout.

Already it was nearly a month since I'd begun walking to the Leverett Circle pedestrian overpass. I was getting better, going farther, building up stamina, but I still needed the railing. Someday, somehow, I'd wean myself from it, just not yet.

My toe still caught on the walkway far more often than permissible for running without the railing. And my gait still didn't feel consistent enough. It just didn't feel ready. Besides, my distance wasn't there yet. I needed to be able to run several miles comfortably before I went off the railing.

All right, enough lazing around. Time to get going.

LOOKING OVER MY SHOULDER AT THE NEIGHBORHOOD as I stretched both Achilles tendons on the front stoop, I noticed that although it was a few hours later than I usually got out, things were quieter in the North End than even I was used to. On-street parking, usually bumper to bumper, wasn't. All over the neighborhood, people must have already left for Thanksgiving. Walking along the North Station area, I noticed the absence of trucks. Apparently not so many delivered on Thanksgiving.

Not a bad morning for running. The sky looked like rain later on, and it was a bit brisk, but there wasn't much wind. Wind could be the deal breaker to a run this morning.

As winter approached, I sometimes wondered if I'd keep running. through the cold. It wasn't the actual running. While I ran, the exertion kept me plenty warm, sometimes too warm, sweating even. It was walking over to Leverett Circle and then walking home after sweating. How was I going to handle it when it got really cold? But right now it was only Thanksgiving and technically still autumn. I'd deal with winter when it came. Or maybe I'd get lucky and it'd be a warm one.

Walking toward Leverett Circle, I noticed my walking felt different—better somehow, reminiscent even, almost familiar. I tuned in to the observation, concentrating, trying to figure out what "different" actually meant.

Since the hemorrhage—it would be ten years next June 19—I'd done this countless times. I called it a "concentrated walk." "Concentrated" because of the intense attention I focused on the *whats*, *whys*, and *hows* of each step: What was different? Why was it different? How was I doing it? "Where in me was I doing something or somethings different?"

"Concentrated" also because the distance of the walk was enough to alter and tinker and otherwise work on understanding the way I moved my legs, hips, shoulders—everything, and to give me time to fine-tune what I was noticing.

During "moments of brilliance" like this one, times when my gait felt better, a concentrated walk was walking long enough for me to attempt to seize the body memory of what felt better, to capture a kinesthetic understanding of what was working at that moment, to try secure an awareness of the sequences, to capture in my memory the movements in my neck, shoulders, scapulae, arms, spine, ribs, hips, thighs, knees, calves, ankles, heels, and toes—everyehere, and the synergies among all the muscles and ligaments linking my bones together.

Every other day, walking from my apartment to Leverett Circle was yet another opportunity for a concentrated walk, should there be a moment of brilliance. With no one around to speak to me, no one to keep pace with, with negligible traffic on the streets and sidewalks. I could focus on myself with the necessary heightened awareness.

With my walking feeling better this Thanksgiving morning I concentrated on "better." How was it better? More even? I listened inside and outside, concentrating. I directed my focus, noticing how my movement felt and how it sounded. As I'd imagined before getting up, the sound of walking wasn't only my footsteps but also the rubbing of material against material, of my hair against material, and the breeze across my ears. I listened to it all.

I walked this morning with a purpose, with a direction and a destination, not dawdling. But that wasn't the difference. In the early morning, I always walked briskly over to Leverett Circle. Yet this morning, something about my gait felt vaguely familiar. Another of Feldenkrais practitioner Mia Segal's remarks echoed in my head: "Tommye?" She'd always spoken my name as if it were a question. "Move your behind. You must attract attention." I'd laughed self-consciously, wondering what in the world she was talking about and thinking Me? Attract attention? Who in the world would pay attention to human wreckage like me? I'd rejected the idea as ridiculous. My hemi-paretic body no longer had the movse to "attract attention." I remembered thinking.

Having said it, Mia never revisited the thought, as if it were enough to have planted it in my mind. With her decade old words echoing in my mind, I reached around behind me, resting the inside of my wrist against the small of my back, my fingers loosely curled Was that part of it? The description for what I felt came to mind as "Broken Away," a separateness I didn't remember noticing before—movement between my lumbar vertebrae, tailbones and my behind.

I opened my hand, spreading it thumb to pinkie finger across my buttocks, the heel of my hand over my tailbones. Umm, yes, there seemed to be movement, as if the four bone structures (my two way lower vertebrae and both halves of my pelvis) which I remembered having moved as one, as if fused together—by the stroke? by spasticity? by neural impulses I no longer knew how to send?—had unfused.

Why today did I feel each a separate bone yet moving in concert with the others—connected together but distinct? What was different? What had allowed these bones to articulate, separating from one another? Or perhaps a better question: Now that it was happening, now that my spine and pelvis seemed to have broken away from one another, how would it reflect in my running? Thinking about that, I wished I didn't have to waste my hand holding onto the railing as I ran. I wished I could leave my hand right here, feeling whether there was still articulation as I ran.

I walked past closed bars, restaurants, and lone strip joints that wouldn't open until at least noon—quite a while yet. A little farther down, the McDonald's, Burger King, and Seven-Eleven would be ringing up sales, but nothing along this stretch. Perfect conditions for listening.

The city had recently installed wide, smooth sidewalks, with hardly any "cracks to break your mother's back." The childhood rhyme made me smile, though with a wave of sadness over the loss of my childhood ableness. After almost a decade, my childhood seemed almost like someone else's childhood, or as if it were a vividly recalled past life from which I'd reincarnated.

Still, my left foot seemed quieter this morning—the footstep firm but not slapping the pavement. That was good but not exactly revolutionary. During other "moments of brilliance," I'd sometimes heard quietness when my left foot reached for the ground.

Reached. That was an interesting word to describe walking. Why had I thought it? Arms reach, hands reach, but feet and legs? And yet, that was it. I listened harder, listening inside my body, inside my legs, focusing and concentrating. How did legs reach? I listened way up high past my buttocks, to where my hand still rested, straddling lumbar vertebrae in my lower back, my ileum, sacrum, and coccyx, my tailbones, and down my legs to my feet, in ankle bones, heel bones, my metatarsals, my phalange. I listened to my hamstrings, to my quadriceps, and to the stretching in the backs of my knees.

Stretching in my knee—that would happen with reaching, wouldn't it? Though still not as even as a metronome, I listened to my footsteps, sounding more alike on the cement sidewalk. I moved determinedly toward Leverett Circle. Yet my steps seemed longer and looser.

Longer. That was the familiarity. It had to be. Inside, my stomach did the cartwheel-off-the-high-beam-bounce-and-present that it used to do when my team won a hard-played game against a strong opponent. A flip so forceful, for a moment I thought I might throw up.

I'd been tall all my life, reaching my full five feet eight inches when I was twelve years old and in the sixth grade. My smaller friends had walked a step and a half, or two sometimes, to my one stride. Even girls my height hadn't taken such long, limber strides—perhaps it wasn't ladylike. I never knew. But long and limber had felt good, powerful. On campus at Wheaton, the sound of my heels clack-clacking across the linoleum tiles of the halls, over carpet-covered hardwood corridors, sounded controlled and safe. In New York, along city sidewalks crowded with people, my determined stride carried me through. In subway tunnels, at night, my no-nonsense, firm and powerful "I know where I'm going" gait protected me. I'd liked the clack-clack my heels made, a measured, steady, firm tat-tat, tat-tat of an in-control, "don't mess with me" woman.

That was the me I'd lost when blood vessels in my brain hemorrhaged. Was I relearning it? getting my "me" back? Or at least starting to? So it seemed.

Was it my right leg allowing my left to reach out longer as well as change in my left leg? Was looseness related to the "breaking away" of the bones in the small of my back and below? The "why" and "how" seemed important. My experience was that change tended to be a combination of "*whys*" and "*hows*," a complicated commingling of variables allowing change to happen.

More important was focusing on the sensations, on implanting the changes in my conscious and subconscious mind, to understand and remember the synergies between my bones, muscles, tendons, and ligaments, the synergies that had allowed this to happen. I looked up, aware now of the streets around me.

Oh my God. I caught my breath. How did I get here? The

silent question in my mind accusing. Slowly I scanned the streetscape around me. I recognized all the landmarks, the buildings, the shuttered stores, the Emerson Lane Fortuna building, renovated not long ago, with its already tarnished bronze statues of scantily draped female forms out front. It was all en route to Leverett Circle.

But how? I searched my mind, more and more afraid. How did I get this far without noticing? I should remember crossing a main street, shouldn't I? I wouldn't have stepped off the curb and across to the center island and across more traffic lanes without remembering. Still I walked on toward my destination, trying to concentrate on the longer looseness of my gait, but worried, too.

Since I was six or seven years old, I'd been crossing streets alone, cautiously and safely looking both ways. Surely I'd remember. I scanned what surrounded me again. How could I have gotten here without knowing it? I remembered walking out the side door of the condominium into the alley, down the alley onto Thacher, and left onto Endicott. I remembered crossing Cross Street and then North Washington to the Haymarket bus plaza, up to the crosswalk, and across New Chardon to Canal Street. How did I remember every step of the way except . . . I looked around me again.

WELL, OF COURSE. THE BOTTOM FALLING OUT IN MY stomach. I hadn't gotten to Causeway Street. I hadn't crossed it yet. It was a wave of relief—but of dread, too. How was it possible I could have been so confused? How did a cerebral hemorrhage take away spatial orientation? Intellectually, I acknowledged the loss and understood my confusion, yet the desire to collapse into a fetal squat, hugging my knees weeping uncontrollably, almost overwhelmed.

The hemorrhage had reduced my world to an unconnected, unrelated tableau of landmarks, disconnected snapshots that so often fit together unexpectedly. Sometimes I got thinking about something else, if I wasn't paying attention to what surrounded me, like this morning, the snapshots got shuffled.

Ordinarily, I was paying attention and wasn't so inwardly focused. Ordinarily, I was confident of my physical safety.

Oh, hell, I thought, no harm done. Nothing accomplished by wasting time brooding over once being able to scan around me, think a moment, and just know where I needed to be. If I kept going, maybe I'd still have my lower back and pelvis broken away. Maybe I wouldn't lose the change, only to regain it sometime in the future maybe—the unpredictable progression of rehabilitation . . .

Causeway Street was now just over the curb, and I still had a run to fit in before Thanksgiving dinner and before the rain. The gray sky overhead looked more and more troubled.

Last night's rain still mottled the cement sidewalks with dampness. The high-school football fields were already soggy, so no use hoping it wouldn't rain before the Thanksgiving games. My goal was to finish up the outside stuff—running and traveling to my folks—between showers.

I stepped onto the cement walkway after stretching my Achilles on the stairs. Despite "getting lost," it still felt like a good day for running—not such a great day for photographs, but I hadn't come for "pics," and my leg just felt good.

I glanced at my watch. I'd taken far too long walking over here. There were only a couple ways to cram more exercise into a morning: get here faster or run the route faster. I was up to three laps, but how far was a lap? I had no clue how far I was running.

Crossing the walkway at the end of the third lap, I glanced at my watch. I'd pushed these laps a bit faster. Good. That was the plan. My breathing was still easy. I could go for a fourth, no problem.

I turned, facing up the ramp, my right hand again resting on the handrail. After three laps, my legs seemed to be getting the idea. This time, the rocking felt only minimally necessary—back and forth a couple of times, and I was off.

Starting up the ramp toward the first curve, I focused my listening on those bones at the end of my spine, to where they fit into my pelvis, on the ligaments and tendons connecting those bones and on whether they'd retained the flexibility I'd noticed while walking. Without being able to touch that place with my hand, it was hard to be certain.

As I'd come to the end of the third lap, my legs felt as though they could keep going and still have enough left for the walking and standing I needed to do. I could feel the effort I was expending in my butt, my gluteus maximus, both left and right, though more in the left. What was different today? Different was change, and, in my experience with rehab, change was good. It might not be better now, but with time, with change somewhere else and somewhere else, it could be. At least it suggested change was still possible.

Enough changes in the right directions and I'd be running free, anywhere I wanted, no longer needing this stupid handrail, my hand free to wipe sweat from my brow, hold a tissue and blow my nose, and to rest against the small of my back or my stomach, feeling my muscles.

Starting the fourth lap, I considered maybe even running a fifth . . . Later in the afternoon I could rest, after dinner. Crossing the walkway at the other end, I set out up the ramp for the fourth return pass over Leverett Circle. I'd seen only a few people crossing the walkway this morning, and I'd just completed half a lap more than I'd run before. Starting the uphill bit again, I felt the added effort, but still my legs felt good. I had to pay attention to this second half of the fourth lap—make sure it didn't get sloppy. Maybe I should coach myself out loud.

With all the people I'd been sharing the overpass with, I'd stopped coaching myself out loud. Talking to myself seemed to make people uneasy. Besides, it probably looked weird enough, a woman running around and around a pedestrian walkway, without talking too. Today though, I had the place to myself, and even if I didn't, coaching out loud felt like the right thing to do.

"Keep going, keep going, no slackin'. Come on, kid. Reach-and, reach-and, reach-and." I kept my voice low and deep, coming from well below my vocal cords, and chanted steadily. "Step out, mmmm, step-out, thatsa-girl. B'llet foot, b'llet foot. Heel first, heel first, come on, come on, heel first, heel first. Reach-and, reach-and.

"Tommye? You must attract attention." Mia's remembered words overlay my chant like lyrics with a beat. "Come on, come on. Atta girl. Keep it goin', keep it goin'." "You must attract attention."

On and on I ran, chanting, to the end of the walkway, around and back up. My right leg felt fine; plenty left for a fifth lap. The left one felt unusual— "hollow" was the word that came to mind. Whatever that meant. I could hear my footsteps, still asymmetrical. Though my stride felt almost nothing like "real" running, this morning, running was just feeling better. Even if my left leg felt detached in its effort at the moment and I wasn't aware of muscles, bones, or anything else inside it, I was still conscious of my foot. I could feel it landing on the walkway. I could still feel my weight ride through the step and push off into the next stride. I knew my ankle was straining to flex and extend the way it was supposed to. Straining because I still didn't have the fluidity in my ankle to ride my foot through its natural range of motion.

"Reach-and, reach-and, reach-and, reach-and." Crossing the walkway to begin another lap, I continued encouraging myself out loud still thinking Yes, I am going to push for that fifth go-round.

Starting up the walkway, I concentrated on the sounds—my left foot hitting the pavement, on the almost inaudible rubbing of my nylon suit—and focused on the momentum from my right leg guiding each stride. Listening to running wasn't unusual, but this time around, how it sounded would be my main source of information about my left leg.

From experience with a paralyzed leg, I knew not being able to feel it wasn't as serious as it might sound. "Not feeling" seemed to be a function of over stimulating the leg, of pushing hard. I could remember it happening when I'd skied farther than I had before, or maybe on the first run after time off. It could happen walking a long way—home from the Boston Public Library in Copley Square for example.

Not being able to feel my leg had yet to precede injury of any kind, so I didn't worry about "hollowness." I just observed. It occurred to me this was what it would feel like if body parts could be hypnotized while the mind remained clear. As long as I attended to my running, listened closely, and felt my foot and ankle, I'd be fine.

"Go on, go on, keep goin', keep goin'. You're doin' fine. Keep goin', keep goin'." I talked myself along. Back down to street level at the Esplanade, four and a half laps completed, I crossed the walkway, heading back to the beginning, and watched as heavy, cold raindrops stained the cement. Rain ruled out any thought I might have had about walking the second half of this fifth lap. We're going to get wet, kids, I told myself, but we're going to get wet running.

I could have quit at four laps and, if I had, I'd have been nearly home by the time the rain started. But with this much rain, I'd have gotten soaked anyway. Damn it, it felt better to get wet running, after so many years of accepting a drenching by rain while walking through it. Running—and being able to—felt like taking action, like responding to the rainfall.

STEPPING OUT OF THE SHOWER INTO THE LIVING ROOM, wrapped in my terrycloth robe, I flopped down on the floor, my legs in a straddle, left foot pressed flat against the wall, to stretch for the second time in one morning. Five laps, the cold rain, and the standing around I'd be doing later merited another stretch.

Probably I should think about fitting in another one yet, perhaps shortly after I got to my folks' house, before people started coming, and again maybe between the cocktail party and dinner, and even after dinner. The bus, all that sitting—dinner and gabbing—and the standing around, would be perfect opportunities for my muscles to seize up uncomfortably. It wasn't exactly painful, the spastic tone in my left side—but rather a low-grade irritant making my movement less fluent. Since the plan was to somehow teach my muscles to get over their spastic status quo and learn to participate in activities the rest of the world enjoyed, without my having to think about each step of every activity, preventative stretching was in order.

Fourteen:
Friday after Thanksgiving

OUTSIDE NORTH STATION, WEARING A HERRINGBONE tweed suit under my long champagne-white nylon overcoat, and my briefcase packed full and slung across my chest, I waited for the gray Boston Coach van to take me to work at the World Trade Center. Just out of the rain I rocked side to side, my feet shoulder-width apart.

What was the deal with that right gluteus muscle in my butt? Each sway of my hip over the right little-toe side of my foot, I felt the strain. Mmm there it is, that's good, that's good, lean into it, I told myself silently. What had I done differently yesterday, except go farther? After running, I'd lingered in the shower so much longer than normal and puttered around, taking my time getting dressed, until finally catching a later bus than I'd planned. When I got to the house, people were already arriving. I'd thought I'd have plenty of time to stretch before all the standing around. Instead, I went straight from sitting on the bus for forty-five minutes and walking half a mile, to standing around gabbing and eating hors d'oeuvres for a couple of hours, to sitting down to Thanksgiving dinner and then joining those watching the games on TV. That was probably it.

Luckily, I'd had running to talk about since work wasn't terribly exciting. Aunt Cath's face lit up like a co-conspirator as I told her what I was doing. When my sister heard our cousin Natalie, a YMCA program director, exclaim, "Tommye, you're running? That's so excellent!" Ann crossed her arms high and tight, leaning against the refrigerator between Natalie and me, saying only, "What are you wearing for shoes? You can get really hurt if you don't have good shoes."

I raised my eyebrows, only a bit caught off-guard, and laughed. "I have a pair of Asics. They're fabulous. Great cushion, support, and it feels like walking on air."

"Asics are good running shoes," Nat confirmed, nodding. Ann had turned, joining another conversation before Natalie's questioning for details on the hows and whys.

"HEY! YOU JUST GOING TO STAND THERE, OR ARE YOU GOING out to the World Trade this morning?" Paul leaned across the passenger seat and hollered through the side window of the Boston Coach van.

"Oh, yeah. Hi Paul." I reached for the door handle and opened the front door. Over the months of commuting to the not easily accessed World Trade Center, I'd learned the easiest seat for me to get into was the front. Reaching up, I hooked my fingertips into the gutter over the door, stepped onto the running board with my right foot. Hoisting myself between my right arm and leg, I pivoted into the seat. After so much practice, I felt almost graceful boarding the van.

THERE WAS A DIFFERENT FEEL THIS MORNING IN THE cubicle village where I worked. While the stock market was open—the Friday after Thanksgiving wasn't a Wall Street holiday—volume would likely be light.More had taken the day off than had come in. It was almost quiet in the huge room, the length of a skyscraper toppled on its face, with so many of the cubicles empty. Noticibly absent were the background hum, of discrete conversation, telephones ringing, computer terminals, and keyboards clicking.

Settled into my workstation, I saw only Suzanne in the department, but she was more than a bishop's move away. I worked in silence, studying page after page of account history, trying to understand why an adjustment had deducted several thousand dollars out. It was the accountholder's question too. My job was to find the answer and, if an error, to have the adjustment reversed. With so few people in, I could focus on this problem without having to consult on "items" belonging to my less experienced coworkers, and then I'd tackle the next "item" on my list.

The answer just wasn't in the history. I'd been back and forth through it, and there wasn't any like sum coming in to balance the deduction. Okay. I'd have to hike down to the other end of the room and pull the backup.

I gathered my file in its folder, stuck a post-it note with the critical details on top, and set off on the trek to the other end. Along the way, so few people were in, and only a few of those people I'd met. Just a nod and a "Morning" were necessary as I strode past empty cubicles and then one occupied by an unfamiliar someone.

I was movin'—going faster than anyone there had ever seen me. My bangs bounced against my forehead, and the little hairs on the side of my face fluttered tickling the skin.

Wrong aisle, I thought, laughing to myself. I'd misjudged. The lateral file drawers I needed to rummage through for the adjustment back-up were in the aisle to my right. Like a quarter horse rounding up a steer, I lost no speed as I smoothly cut around to the space between cubicles where—Uh! I didn't see it knee-high, tucked against Michael's cubicle wall.

My left foot struck the stack of computer printouts and I was airborne. Out of the corner of my eye, I saw Michael and two adjustments coworkers spin around in their desk chairs, helplessly watching me thrust myself over the stack, cushioning my landing with a deep knee bend on my right foot before hop-hop-hopping.

Balanced, I swept my right arm in front and around to the side, palm up, the file folder like a baton, in perfect balance-beam dismount form I smiled triumphant and relieved. Around me they stared silently, all three of them, Michael working his jaw, his lips parting and closing wordlessly.

I laughed, breaking the silence, "A ten, right?"

"Jesus, Tommye," Michael exclaimed, words finally coming. "I thought we were going to be picking you off the floor in pieces. You're really okay?"

"Sure." I laughed. "So now that I have your attention . . ." I fanned the file folder, softly fluttering it, "I need to see back-up for this adjustment, so I can explain it to the customer."

A short, round, middle-aged woman I'd not met before stood beside me, her hand on my forearm. " I'm Mary," she said shaking her head. "I've never seen anything like that." She shugged, looking over at Michael and his adjustments coworkers. "Have you?" She turned further to face the windows and those few other heads peering over cubicle dividers.

SETTLING BACK INTO MY DESK CHAIR, PREPARING TO write an explanation of the adjustment for my customer, I felt the twinge from my right gluteus again, the one I'd noticed earlier. Without the running, I thought, they would have been picking me up in pieces down there.

So maybe it really was worth getting up at four in the morning . . .

Fifteen:
Going Out

I'D RUSHED HOME, AND PUSHED THROUGH MY STRETCHING and strengthening physical therapy floor exercises—the protocol I did every afternoon—hurrying, because tonight I was going to the company Christmas party. A gala affair of too much alcohol, ice sculptures filled with jumbo shrimp, dancing, laughter, and talk with employees company-wide.

Last year when they held it at the World Trade Center, the building was still the partially renovated, cavernous former shipping warehouse. We'd milled around on cement floors looking at gray construction mats hung along the walls for insulation and wandered through the massive, drafty, garage-like rooms in party clothes no one saw, because we never took off our overcoats. I'd kept thinking about those poor people who'd had to work out there rather than in company properties downtown, and now, six months later, I was just another one of those exiled to the pier, the World Trade Center.

This year, the World Trade Center was still cavernous, but the ceilings were finished, the floors carpeted, and we'd be hanging up our coats since they'd hooked up the heating system. Tonight, the building would be dressed up for a company-wide party on three floors.

I hadn't planned to wear anything special—just a suit or regular work clothes—until I saw what my coworkers had brought with them to change into. Instead of going home, getting ready and coming back, they'd decided to put in a few hours of overtime, theoretically getting more work done before getting dressed for the party.

One look at what Sue, Kathy, Eileen, and women in other departments had brought to wear convinced me a suit just wouldn't do—not this year—these were real cocktail party dresses. Once home, I pulled the "café au lait" cocktail dress Gram and I had found for me in Florida out of the closet to look at it. I wasn't the oldest in the department, Carol was a mom with kids graduating college, but I was the only one who was "different." Some of my co-workers, not long out of college, an still lived with their parents. Maybe tonight would be the opportunity to dent their image of me. It felt as though they saw me as so much older, like a glass window they looked right through, with out really seeing.

It wasn't that I wanted to pal around with my coworkers. I just hoped for a feeling of congenial friendliness. Not that a dress or a company party could actually retool an image people seemed to have of me, but maybe it could scratch up the glass some.

Clad only in my nylons, I slid the dress off its hanger. In a moment, it was over my head, set on my shoulders, the sleeves adjusted, and the front hook fastened. I smoothed only a touch of makeup onto my face and some lipstick before checking the effect in the full-length mirror tacked to the back of the closet door.

Umm, I looked good in that dress, the wide-belted waist accentuating a slender figure I never thought of myself as having, the way no business suit ever could, or should. And the demure, almost Nehru neck, clasped just below the notch in my collarbone, only hinted at the slit down the front to the belted waist.

I turned side to side two, maybe three times, taking it in. Was this really me? My hair, newly cut, hugged my head "just like a cap," as Aunt Kitty had exclaimed when she saw me last. My shoulders, still broad, strong, and even, despite the hemi-paresis had, never needed the padding that was all the rage now Oh, get over it, I thought, raising my eyebrows, still looking at my reflection before I scrunched my eyes lips, and cheeks making one of those faces Gram had always chided me about.

I rarely looked at myself in a full-length mirror—especially dressed for a cocktail party—and it surprised me that I looked better than I had in college. Right there in front of me I saw me firmer, stronger, and thinner. The running? Glancing down at the hem, I realized quite a bit more leg showed than my suits allowed. Oh, Gram, I thought, you wild one, you. The dress had been her choice that day.

My wristwatch beeped the hour . . . time traveled on. Seven had seemed an appropriate time to leave so I'd arrive fashionably late. I threw on my coat. I wouldn't need a wallet—just some money, in case I needed a cab home, and my employee ID, to get into to the party.

For no reason other than variety, I'd decided to catch one of the Fidelity shuttles from State Street rather than the regular van from North Station. I was feeling good. Walking out of my place. I noticed my stride felt looser and more confident—more "normal."

I looked forward to seeing people I'd worked with before transferring around. Hey, I got around better than I had then—I was better—almost passing for normal now.

Ugh, I thought, stepping out onto the street. Seven o'clock, and already it's pitch black dark. At least there were the Christmas lights, a bit of not-soot-covered snow, and the city street lights. Even on a frosty, wintry evening, other people were out walking after dark. People always walked in the North End: residents, visitors, and tourists. Always.

I hadn't been to this end of Prince Street for quite a while—North Square, with its huge Christmas tree in the center of the cobblestone island in front of Mamma Maria's. It was perfect. I walked slower, taking it in. This was what made Christmas special, lighting the dark of night with color.

"Excuse me, can I ask you a question?"

I'd just turned onto North Street when a twenty-something blonde caught up to me, butting her head around from my left. I slowed more, realizing as I did how much of the looseness and confidence my stride lost in the slowing.

"Um, I was walking behind you, and maybe this is rude, but I'm kinda drunk, and I thought it was ruder to wonder and not ask."

I stared at her, trying to guess her question. It didn't sound as though she were trying to find one of the restaurants, the Old North Church, Paul Revere's House, where she'd parked her car, or the subway . . . Those were the questions visitors and tourists usually asked. I waited, fighting the urge to check my watch—after all, I did have a place to go and people to meet, and I was almost looking forward to this party.

Astonishingly, tonight of all nights, her question was "Why do you limp?"

I turned slowly my whole body, so not only my eyes faced her, and shook my head. How do I answer? Grab her by the shoulder and shake some sense in? Shout that she's a stupid insensitive bitch? Just tell her—reaching inside and feeling the hurt all over again? What for? Who the hell was she to me?

"I mean, I was wondering, what happened, you know, that you walk with a limp?"

My head cocked to the left, I opened my eyes even wider holding them fixed on hers, knowing full well how it would look to her. Softly and oh so calmly, I replied, "That has got to be the most insensitive, most immature, most unimaginative question I have ever been asked."

"Well, I thought it was ruder for me to walk along behind you, wondering."

Lowering my eyebrows, I began to speak again, my head still tipped to the side. "You know, that's what's wrong with you twenty-somethings. You've lived your lives with everything explained for you—videos on TV, or pumped into your heads through Walkman headsets." I shook my head, my eyes still locked on hers. "You have no imagination." I paused. "What if you could make up an explanation of your own, a story explaining it for yourself?"

She stared at me blankly.

I continued, "what if you imagined me driving with my fiancé and we were way out going to meet his family. And, coming down the long hill before turning off to the house, the brakes failed? What if you imagined my fiancé struggling to regain control." I waited.

"But the tree. What if you imagined he died and I lived, and so now you imagine that still, after how many surgeries, I limp. And I always will. Each step reminding me."

She reached as if to touch my shoulder, her lips pressed together and twisted the way I knew they would when the credits filled the screen after a tragic love story like Dr. Zhivago. I shifted away from her, leaving her hand to reach for the air separating us.

"Oh, I'm sorry." Her voice appropriately soft and empathetic. "Is that why?"

I raised my eyebrows again, fighting the urge to laugh. "Maybe," I smiled, still oh so calm, so controlled. "Or maybe you can come up with a better story." I turned away from her, saying, "But right now, I'm running late." And I had to get back to remembering how confident I'd felt, how confident in how I looked and in how I would present at the company party.

I stepped away, conscious of how standing still for just those few moments had caused the joints on my left side to tighten up—as if, in standing those minutes, they forgot how to make my leg walk, emphasizing the limp. Come on, kids, I told myself silently. She'll be watching you walk away. Do it with confidence and skill and no limp, I told myself. It was a valid goal, at least. Some day I'd get there. Someday I really would "pass for normal." Someday people would stop asking what was wrong with me and would be back to trying to figure out what was so right.

I never looked back to see if she watched. But in case she did, and even more for me, as I passed Paul Revere's House I laughed out loud and loudly. Limp! I thought, laughing. That girl should have seen me when they first stood me between the parallel bars, a leather strap around my waist and two physical therapists hanging tight, my right hand clinging to the bar on the right. This was nothing.

Eat your heart out, babe.

Sixteen:
Christmas Morning

ALL MY GIFTS WERE WRAPPED. I HAD CHRISTMAS PILED HIGH on my living room floor, waiting to be packed up and hauled to my folks' on the bus. Kate, my brother's daughter and my first niece, was almost a year and a half old. She'd be our Christmas child, making it fun this year. Last year, Christmas was a bunch of grownups standing around giving each other festively wrapped gifts with not-even-five-month-old Kate wailing in my brother's arms—the break from her normal routine proving to be too much to handle.

I imagined that this morning, nobody'd be around to witness my first annual Christmas run. Surely everyone but me was already home for the holidays, especially with Christmas and Chanukah overlapping this year. I'd stayed in town for

Christmas Eve, to be with friends and so I could get in a long, early-morning run, wearing my Christmas present to myself.

Oh, big deal, I thought. A terrycloth sweatband. Yeah, but a true fashion statement—lime green to match the panels at the shoulders on my running suit. Yeah, the fashion goddess, whatever her name, would so approve—if she hadn't fallen over in a dead faint at the thought of a color-coordinated me.

As I stretched, I thought about the Christmas plans. After I arrived at my folks' and we exchanged our presents, we were off to my brother and sister-in-law and Kate's house to exchange presents with them and Ann and my brother-in-law. And for brunch.

Mmm, all that good food—blueberry cake, different quiches, the honey ham that seemed to be all the rage these days, probably Mom's raisin bread—the envy of all my friends growing up—maybe Aunt Kitty's Stollen . . . hmm, what else? I had such an appetite these days. Food never used to be particularly important to me—maybe the running?

But brunch would be a perfect reward for the eight laps I had planned for my Christmas 1990 morning nine years, six months, and six days after the hemorrhage.

Last time out, I'd counted the paces in a lap around the overpass and back. Seven hundred forty. At a conservative two feet per pace, I was running 1,480 feet per lap. Times eight laps was 11,840 feet, about two and a quarter miles. So, I thought, eleven laps would be a touch over three miles. In not too long, that would be my distance . . .

But even with practice and more distance, periodically there'd be that kkrhrrh, scraping of my left toe catching on the walkway. It was better than in the beginning, when with nearly every stride, my left foot caught on the cement. Yet it happened often enough the handrail still seemed necessary.

How did I fix that? I pondered, pressing my forehead into my left knee. What did I have to do to make the synergy—ankle/knee/hip-flex—as automatic as the knee/hip-flex/flaccid ankle was now? I kept working on it. Standing still anywhere—waiting for a subway train, for a "walk" signal, to meet a friend, or just in line, I'd rock forward and back, my feet a pace apart, left in front. That should help reinforce the flex/flex/flex synergy I needed to make automatic in my running and my walking gaits.

Someday fairly soon, I needed to be ready to wean myself from that walkway. As perfect as it was for teaching myself to run, it already felt líke another hamster wheel, prison-like, and oh, too familiar. By now, I knew every crack along the way, every defect in the railing. I practically recognized the cars commuting through the rotary every morning. Me . . . the one who might remember if someone's car had two or four doors and maybe whether it was blue or white, but the make? Me, recognizing cars . . . it was absurd.

Starting on my way over for my Christmas run on the hamster wheel—What nonsense, I reprimanded myself. Running was fun, I found myself fighting the desire to turn around and go back to bed.

I should have known to get myself to sleep earlier last night. Stupid, foolishness—staying up so late. Going back to bed seemed infinitely preferable to walking, what, three-quarters of a mile dressed in this nylon suit with a thin cotton-poly fleece lining, in weather cold enough to see my breath, and a light dusting of snow almost crunching underfoot. The sweatband over my ears helped some, and once I got running there'd be plenty of body heat—but walking over . . . especially today. Walking over seemed more than a body should have to endure.

Yes, and how do you expect to teach yourself to run if you crawl back into bed just because you're a little tired and it's a little cold out? the parent voice in my head demanded.

It was true. If I once let myself just not feel like running once, it would happen again and again, until . . . No, there could be no turning back. There'd be no first time. Someday, somehow, I was going to learn how to get off that handrail, so I could run where I pleased—whenever I pleased. I just wasn't ready yet. I'd know when I was ready. With my toe still scraping the pavement kkrhrrh, often enough that without the railing I'd be forever picking myself up off the street, causing traffic incidents, I wasn't ready yet.

Whenever I was out walking and fell—it happened enough to remember, more these days, now that I was walking differently, walking harder and faster, with more involvement in my hips, lower back, and shoulders, more involvement everywhere—someone driving by would pull over, jump out of their car or even big rig truck, and rush over to help me up. I needed to wait until I was pretty sure I would-n't fall. Besides, the point of teaching myself to run was to stay on my feet and get cardiovascular exercise in the company of others, not to find a new way to scrape even more skin off my body and upset innocent passersby.

I walked through a city decorated for the holidays and delighting with its festivity. This early in the morning, the sky still dark, the lights pinpoints against the night, a dusting of snow festively covering even the electric wires between the colored bulbs, the wires not carefully hidden behind the city-sized pine-bough wreaths hanging in commercial building doorways or decorating expanses of wall, wreaths as big around as I was tall, with red-ribbon bows scaled to fit.

The early-morning quiet echoed with the crunch of new snow underfoot. Softly, softly, like a music box I might have had as a child, I heard the clear one-by-one metallic notes to "Silent Night." In my mind I heard the German lyric to those notes, the way Chas presented them to us in freshman choir.

You would have missed this private holiday moment to go back to bed, I chided myself. You can sleep any time of the year. But this, this is a life experience—something to tell the grandchildren about. Of course, I'd need at least one child before I could tell grandchildren anything.

Rounding the corner finally to where the overpass emptied onto the sidewalk in front of that funny slate blue building, I glanced around. It wasn't all that decorated over here. The spire-like antenna thing on the dome of the Mugar Omni

Theater, unadorned, reached into the sky the way it always did. Perhaps a star perched atop or a big red bow draped over the dome would be too sacred for a Science Museum. But wouldn't it be fun? I'd enjoy looking at it, and how many others too?

I got going right away. It was too cold to stand around just rocking, and I'd walked briskly. A single back-and-forth and I was off. Pick up that leg. Up with the foot. Come on, up, up, I coached myself silently. Heel-toe, heel-toe. My footsteps landed loudly in the early holiday-morning quiet. Even the rubbing of the nylon under my left arm almost echoed. Ooh, it was cold. Crossing the walkway at the Esplanade end, I touched the back of my wrist against my cheeks, one by one, then my nose. I should probably consider wearing that polypropylene face mask I'd used when I skied. It was still in the cabinet by the door, with the rest of my winter stuff. Frostbite on the face wouldn't be a positive outcome to this running project—Mother would never approve.

"You're out here today, too . . . " called out a state trooper, crossing the parking lot. Thinking I was all by myself, I nearly jumped out of my skin. Instead I kept on running. Atta girl, atta girl, I coached my left leg. Keep goin', keep goin' . . . Not even a kkrhrrh from my foot. Good girl . . .

"Don't you take a day off?" He paused in the nearly empty lot, looking up at me.

Apparently he'd seen me out here before—through the station windows, maybe? I couldn't remember ever seeing any state police notice me. I laughed. Where had he come from? A door on the other side of the building?

"Every other day I take off. And this isn't one of them, it's just Christmas," I smiled, still running.

I'd never tried talking while running before—I already knew how problematic talking and walking could be. That was usually when I crashed, when I was paying more attention to gabbing than to walking . . .

"You really work at this . . . "

He was behind me now, until I rounded the corner on the walkway and began tracking back. Pay attention. Kkrhrrh. Oh, damn, there goes that toe. Pay attention to what you're doing, Tomm, I told myself. Up, up, lift up that leg and heel-toe. There you go.

As I rounded the corner, he reached to unlock the cruiser, taking his time, still looking up toward me. "And I'm going to get good at it too." I said, smiling. "Merry Christmas!"

"Ho, ho, ho, and to you." That said, he opened the door, settled into the seat, and started the engine seemingly in one movement before slamming the door shut. Apparently our little chat was over.

Just as well—even that little bit of talking and listening interrupted my concentration. Just as Dad had told his midget football team—boys ten, eleven, twelve years old: "When your mouth's working, nothing else is."

It would be a while before I'd be running with anyone—if

ever. Maybe running would always have to be my thing alone, even though it would be more fun to run with people. Of course, everyone I saw running across the walkway on their way to the Esplanade wore a headset clamped to their heads and a Walkman clipped to a pocket or clenched in a fist.

How did they run without monitoring the sounds of their running and the noises around them? Those runners were so tuned into their Walkmen, they often didn't acknowledge when I nodded and smiled. So actually, there probably wouldn't be much difference between running alone and running with someone else . . .

Okay, okay, you're distracted, I told myself. What're you doing? What're you doing? Where's your weight? Why are you sitting back on your heels? Come on, come on. Get that weight forward, over your toes. Over your toes. Lead with your nose—you're moving forward, not pulling back. That's better, that's better. On both feet, both feet. Lighten up on the handrail. You're not supposed to be leaning, just touching it—barely a "white-glove test." Come on, come on, pay attention. That's it. Lift that leg, bring that foot through. Feel it on the right, copy on the left. Lift with the quads, lift with the lats, lift with the abdominals. Lift with anything that will. Come on, Tomm, "Monkey see, monkey do. Monkey feel, monkey mimic." There you go, there you go, that's better. Clo-opp, clop. Clo-opp, clop. There you go. It's getting there. There you go. It's a little more even. That's better. Push off, push off. Push off.

The warm sweat dripping off my hair cooled quickly on

my neck, dripping down into the collar of my jacket. Each step shifted my jacket, pumping a burst of warm air up from my back and onto my neck. Keep going, keep going. A subway train had just stopped at Science Park station, leaving a handful of Christmas morning travelers on the platform.

Not so many people were traveling as usually did. I hurried to pass where they would enter the walkway. It was a smallish clump of people, but they were heavily laden with parcels—Christmas gifts like the ones I'd soon be hauling on the bus. Even if only two or three of those people were planning to go where I was heading, I'd have to stumble at a walking pace behind them. If they went the other way, perhaps by the time I got to the end of this lap and around to start the next, they'd be enough ahead so there wouldn't be a problem.

Come on, come on keep going, push, push, push. That's a girl. You're doing it, you're doing it.

"Good morning! Merry Christmas," one of the women called out.

I panted, took a deep breath, chanting to myself silently Keep going, keep going, keep going, and smiled, responding with a heartier "Merry Christmas" than I'd intended. The rest of the people seemed to wake up, and we were smiling at one another, wishing each other Merry Christmas. Me? I kept running. This was nearly the seventh lap—one more and home. My legs felt okay. Eight weren't going to be too much. I'd still have enough left to do Christmas with the family.

"Looking good," another runner called out to me as she

passed, running beautifully. I kept running, following her, though dropping farther and farther behind. What did she do? What was she doing differently? I kept watching even as she melted into the early morning duskiness.

Pushing, came the answer. Pushing. I watched her stride roll smoothly through her feet, pushing down through the arch, propelling her forward. Even as she faded from clear view, I could see how her body weight pushed forward through her feet, her legs, her haunches, torso, and arms. She ran fluidly, even rounding the corner. While I still had her in sight, I tried fix in my mind how she looked. I wanted the memory of what moving that way looked like, someday I'd copy how she looked, By imagining I'd know how it would feel. Even after she'd gone so far ahead as to be out of sight, while still running I continued fixing in my mind how she had looked, trying to remember in my body how my legs would feel, my feet, my shoulders.

Keep on going, keep on going. You're doing fine. You're doing better. Keep it going, keep it going. That's a girl, atta girl. Come on, come on. I stepped off the walkway, letting go of the handrail just as the sky began to lighten—time to be finishing up.

It was supposed to be an overcast day, threatening snow but never actually producing . . . Lucky for us, Kate was probably too young to understand that Santa was supposed to arrive in a sleigh pulled by reindeer—and he couldn't have gotten here last night without snow. If she did question, her parents were responsible for coming up with some sort of excuse. Though if pressed, I could probably come up with a "McGivered" story to satisfy her for another year . . .

IN A COUPLE OF HOURS I'D BE LEAVING FOR THE BUS, and I'd have done my two miles. Already it was later than I'd planned. I'd have to figure out how to juggle a bagel and coffee with all those presents on the bus. Otherwise, I might pass out from starvation on the way to my folks' for Christmas, I thought, walking back to my apartment.

Would anyone notice I was walking better? More solidly, more fluidly? Or would the short distances I'd walk inside people's houses camouflage the changes? I hadn't seen family since Thanksgiving.

I shrugged, pressing my lips together, raising my eyebrows, my head tipping to the side, as if my silent conversation with myself, my thoughts and musings, needed body language to be fully understood. Probably not.

With everything else going on—presents, food, the excitement, and with Mom and Dad and most likely Ann and Bob heading north to ski later in the afternoon—probably no one would notice. Unless trained to look, who would make note of minuscule incremental changes in someone's walk . . . and why should they?

Seventeen:
New Year's Day

NEW YEAR'S EVE LASTED LONG AFTER A LASER LIGHT SHOW illuminated the newly re-lit Custom House clock and after Boston's Times Square–style countdown to midnight. It had continued with First Night revelers wandering North End streets hollering "Anthony! Anthony!" (when would the generation that grew up watching a single thirty-second Prince Spaghetti commercial get over it?) and blowing into plastic-horn noisemakers braying like the last wails of mortally wounded beasts. And not far away, City Hall Plaza had been still thick with concerts, ice sculptures, cultural exhibits and demonstrations, and First Nighters just whooping it up hours after midnight.

Dressed to run, I opened the front door to a stoop awash

in trash left behind by those who'd never learned to pick up after themselves and stepped out into eerie quiet. Could I be the only one in Boston not sleeping off a hangover this morning? What a frightening thought . . .

Well, no people and no traffic would make for good, clean air and the privacy to work on improving my running. Sometimes, with people around, I felt as though I had to be polite and acknowledge them. And traffic negotiating the Circle below me diverted concentration from where it should be—my running. It didn't look as though I had to worry about any distractions this morning.

Stepping around beer bottles, I thought, Geez, where were these people brought up, in a barn? I stretched my Achilles, just as I did before every run.

Walking toward Leverett Circle, I shook my head, thinking, and people complained about the Feasts—the weekend block parties celebrating Italian patron saints. At least the Societies cleaned up afterward. Not perfectly, but the neighborhood never looked like this after a Feast. If ever I'd wanted one of those plastic horns, now was my opportunity—they were everywhere, and only once in a while jammed into trash barrels. The rest littered streets, sidewalks, and playgrounds, making this one of those mornings I thought about how nice it would be for some hard-driving rainstorm to pass through washing away the mess left behind.

But it was too cold to rain. Snow would only cover up the mess for a while, and I didn't really want it to snow. So far, no snow had fallen on a running day, and in the twenty-four hours following a snowfall, the city had the roads and side-walks shoveled and plowed well enough that I'd walked to my overpass, running on schedule despite the snowfall. That was one benefit to living in the city. Cambridge and the suburbs around got choked when it snowed. But Boston was always ready and open for business.

I smiled and waved at the police officer driving by. He seemed to have acknowledged me, though it was hard to tell, between the before-sunrise twilight, the hat he wore pulled down over his forehead, and his coat collar covering more of his face. I thought he might be one of the policemen who usu-ally patrolled down by North Station. Quite a few of the reg-ular delivery truck guys—the Globe and Herald, milk and bread, and even trash truck drivers recognized me now and would call out greetings. It always seemed to be men driving the trucks. But not this morning—surely the regular guys got New Years Day off.

Nobody drove the local roads this morning. I could have walked down the middle of the street the whole way to the overpass—but I took the sidewalk . . . And hardly anyone seemed to be converging in Leverett Circle either. As I stepped onto the walkway, I stifled a yawn—I'd been out cel-ebrating New Year's Eve last night too. Feeling rather ho-hum about still running around and around this stupid walk-way, I set off again.

This morning I needed to step up my time and add a twelfth lap to my run, which would make my distance about three point three miles—a little more than 5 kilometers. I'd been doing the math last night: 10K was about 6.2 miles. So I'd be about half way to running the distance of a 10K—like the Bonne Bell. The Bonne Bell was the only area 10K I recalled hearing about from before. As I remembered, it was a women-only run. I'd never done it though.

My feet pounding the ground, I thought, Running the Bonne Bell. I did like the sound of that. What if I could? New Year's was for making resolutions. Why not? If the race were in the spring, I probably wouldn't make it this year. But there was always next spring to train for, and then again, maybe it was in the fall. That's it, I thought, I'm going to run the Bonne Bell. Running along side the handrail, I felt a shiver of excitement humming up my spine, lifting the hairs on the back of my neck and up through my scalp. Running the Bonne Bell—now that was a resolution.

At the end of the pedestrian walkway, where it emptied out to the Charles Street sidewalk, I stopped running to step across the width for the twelfth time this morning and then lay my hand back on the railing. Rocking only once, I got going again.

I could feel the effort in all my muscles. I'd worked them hard this morning. A few more paces and I was already heading up-grade. I ran, my right hand only skimming over the handrail, hardly even touching. Even on the twelfth lap, when my legs should have been tired and my gait getting sloppy, I was doing all right.

A little farther and I was on the flat heading over Leverett Circle intersection toward the T station, finishing up my twelfth lap—half the distance to Running the Bonne Bell—except, of course, I still relied on a handrail I'd have to graduate from sometime. The sole of my left shoe brushed against the walkway, dragging some. But it hadn't caught kkkrrhkkrh on the tip, tripping me up. That was improvement, though I still wasn't consistently picking that left foot up quite high enough, it was closer to being right. Maybe I would be able to run the Bonne Bell whenever it was next scheduled.

Stepping off the walkway, I looked down at one of those plastic noisemaker horns someone had just left lying on the middle of the sidewalk. I pulled back my left foot and gave that horn the hardest kick my leg was capable of, my eyes following the horn as it skittered across the sidewalk until it teetered over the curb into the gutter. Bending over, I reached for the horn and picked it up, carrying it with me until I came to a trash barrel.

Eighteen:
Look at that Ankle Gimbal!

"HI," I SAID, WALKING THROUGH THE DOORWAY INTO DAVID'S office—I'd knocked first. He twisted around in his chair, greeting me. I stepped around stack after stack of paper. David's "creative piles," I called them. Of course, he insisted they were "primary source documents, carefully arranged."

"You look good," David said. "I like that kilt."

"Thank you." I looked around for a chair that wasn't also stacked high with papers. He was obviously in the middle of pulling together a brief, or a response to one, so he had every scrap of information he might need close at hand. About half an hour ago he'd called, saying he was starved and getting out of there for dinner somewhere, did I want to join him?

Giving up on finding an empty chair, I asked, "Are you at a place you can leave? Or did you get yourself in the middle of something new?"

"No, let's go. I have to get out of here."

I hadn't even taken off my coat, only unfastening the snaps in the elevator. "Good, because I'm starved." I combed my fingers through my hair. "Between 'Desert Shield' and the Fed lowering interest rates three-quarters of a point, the market was nuts today."

David looked up from saving and minimizing the open files on his computer, obviously not connecting the significance of the Fed's move or the Gulf action to the work I did.

"They had me on phones all day—got in at six-thirty to try and get something done on my own work. So I was out the door at four-thirty to run this morning . . . "

"Come on, let's go," David said interrupting me as he picked up the Naugahyde portfolio he always carried, stuffing a handful of papers inside. "I'd like to borrow your brain while we eat."

I smiled, rolling my eyes. "Sure, what's left of it. . ." David and I had always hashed over whatever project du jour absorbed his or my attention—whatever one of us was working on or from the world at large. if he hadn't been in the middle of a brief, we might have discussed the new ruling in Michigan against Jack Kevorkian's assisted suicide, F. W. DeKlerk's repeal of some apartheid laws, or, there was always talk of the Allied forces in Kuwait . . .

"They brought food in for us again today." I shook my head frowning.. "But after a couple of weeks of 'Desert Shield' market volatility already, you couldn't pay me to put another slice of European pizza in my mouth. So I had a plate of salad—well, lettuce, three or four tomato wedges, and a hot pepper, all doused in way too much Italian dressing." I laughed. "I need some real food."

"I suppose that means you're not interested in eating at Unos," David said laughing.

At after seven in the evening, we rode the elevator nonstop to the lobby of Sixty State Street. I wiggled my jaw to pop my ears between the third and second floors. At ground, David held his portfolio over the electric eye on the elevator door, holding it open for me.

"Cutting out early tonight, David?" the security guard behind the lobby desk asked.

"I'll be back after we munch some dinner." David said, his laugh sounding punchy, from too little sleep. I was already pushing my way through the revolving door, David soon following.

"What was that about?" I asked.

David turned down State Street. Already he set a fast pace. Accepting the challenge, I matched him step for step.

"He and I were laughing about how great it was to be a lawyer as I waited for a cab to get me home last night at about three in the morning."

I turned to face him and did a double take, still walking forward and matching his pace. "So you were getting to sleep this morning just about as I was climbing out of bed?"

"I guess so. You were really out running at four-thirty?"

David always liked to walk on my right side, so I could see him, he said, since after the hemorrhage I no longer had left peripheral vision. But that way, if we were talking while we walked, and we usually were, I'd have my head turned to face him, leaving me no sight straight ahead, except for a quick glance now and then to check where I was going.

Between the double take and my remark, his question, and my "Damn straight" laughing response, I hadn't glanced soon enough at where I was going to see. Only when I noticed my left foot feeling unstable somehow, as if she were about to get into trouble did I look down, finding my foot perched precariously over an uneven patch of sidewalk. More than half my foot, from the little toe to my second toe, hung over air, my weight supported only by the big-toe edge of my left foot. Yet my ankle hadn't rolled or twisted over my little toe. Instead, it was stabilizing, allowing my foot to hold me upright, "gimbaling," just as it was designed to do.

"Good girl," I said excitedly. "Look, David!" I reached for his arm, clutching his coat to get his attention, then reached down to stroke my ankle, saying out loud, but to myself, "Good girl." I wanted to touch my ankle and feel how it had reorganized to accommodate this problem with the sidewalk, to understand.

"What?" David stood a moment, looking down on me as I now crouched, feeling my ankle and trying to imprint in my body memory how she'd handled this problem.

Reacting to what he saw as a sprained ankle waiting to happen, David grabbed my shoulders. "Here" he said as he pulled me toward him and away from the drop, shifting my body weight off my left foot.

"Na-no," I protested. "Didn't you see? She was doing it right." I'd wanted to freeze the gimbaling feeling in my body memory, so the next time, my ankle would surely know what to do. It was too late now—I'd been "saved." No going back now, I thought. Maybe I could recreate it in my imagination?

How many times since the hemorrhage had a lesser hazard led to an excruciatingly painful roll of my left ankle? It had to be strength and an agility I'd gotten from running. I wasn't "safe" from never turning my ankle, I knew that. Able-bodied people sprained ankles all the time. I could only hope to become not so vulnerable.

Nineteen:
Running Free

HOW MANY LAPS HAD I RUN TODAY? GOING AROUND AND around the same place morning after morning at the same time, it had gotten to the point my mind tended wander, losing count. I'd walked a different route home this morning, a route leading to the ugliest intersection into the North End for a pedestrian. An intersection I regularly avoided.

Pausing at the traffic signal in front of the old Stop & Shop bakery building, I waited for a walk signal. Thinking back on the run, I remembered the sunrise as it unfolded over the Charles River, shining spectacular colors on Financial District office-building windows.

Twelve laps, I remembered, was that runner passing by,

who turned, looking at me, and said, "Keep it up!" Fourteen was the young woman calling out as we passed one another, she walking to the subway station and me not even halfway around that lap saying, "You are such an inspiration." I shook my head remembering now, even stomping my foot in frustration. Uhh, that ridiculous inspiration thing . . . Give me a break. I'm no more an inspiration than I am an Olympic athlete, or a saint . . .

So it had been fifteen laps, because I'd gone around that once more just to prove I wasn't inspirational in the least—hot sweat dripping off the hair curling over my jacket collar, my soaked tee shirt underneath as wringable as the sweatband around my head. I combed my fingers through the hair hanging just over my neck and wiped my hand across the back of my neck. My hair still dripped. I rubbed the dampness into the skin at the nape of my neck. No, not inspirational at all: dripping wet, my breathing ragged, still relying on a handrail, and my uneven footsteps.

But you know . . . I thought, still waiting for the complicated signal pattern to cycle through to the pedestrian light—there was plenty of time just to stand contemplating the run—You know, my legs still feel pretty good. I could have kept going. Of course, my gait was still creative—I knew for sure it wasn't textbook, especially after being labeled inspirational. She'd never have used that word to describe an "able-bodied" runner . . . Maybe someone a bit overweight, someone older or especially young, but not a trim, almost thirty-three year-old female runner . . .

I watched the light change to let me cross. It was an unconventional bootleg route I had to take—across North Washington at the foot of the bridge and then across Commercial, a pedestrian crossing the traffic planners had theoretically factored into traffic-light timing.

But even if my gait wasn't "normal," I thought, stepping out into the first crosswalk. Even if I didn't stride out, my left foot equal to my right. Even if I wasn't fully rolling through the step with my left yet. Even if I wasn't properly pushing off with my left foot onto my right. Even if my run was still choppier than an able-bodied stride. Even so...

Ooooh! It did feel good. Good to be moving faster than ponderously walking and following behind everyone else. Good to be making a headwind of my own, to be pushing back against the air surrounding me. And it was getting better—ever so slowly, but it was getting better. Across Commercial Street, I turned down Prince just before the run-down-looking parking garage—formerly a Brink's property and location of the fabled "Job."

It was Saturday morning, and still early. Looking down the length of Prince Street, I could see no one was out yet, even down by the bakeries and probably not way down, at the end in North Square, either.

Just before Thanksgiving, the city had repaved the whole length of Prince Street—a good and bad development. While cars driving through no longer rattle-rattle, bang-banged bouncing over potholes, the long, smooth, even-hued one-way street, narrowed by the solid line of cars parked at the curb, had become something of a commuter's shortcut raceway from Charlestown to the Financial District. The potholes, while painful to listen to and to drive over, had at least kept speeds down.

Yet they hadn't refinished the sidewalks in probably forever. The cement had been patched and repatched with crumbly asphalt after countless jackhammerings required by probably decades of repair to the water, sewer, gas, electric, telephone, and cable lines serving the solid rows of brick buildings lining either side the street. Walking the sidewalk was tough duty, and after my run this morning, even if I'd felt just a minute ago, I could have kept going, my legs were tired, as they should be. Turning an ankle, and especially my left, would interrupt my schedule for weeks.

I RARELY WALKED THIS END OF THE STREET, AND THE condition of the sidewalk surprised and worried me. It would be too easy to do some serious damage to myself. I should have taken the regular route home. As I surveyed the footing ahead, my eyes strayed over to the smooth, almost-shiny it-was-still-so-freshly-paved street. I already knew hardly anyone was up and out this first Saturday in February.

Why not just walk in the street? Pedestrians did it all the time in the North End. Often, the too-narrow sidewalks for so many getting around on foot, overflowed pedestrians into the streets. The one car that might come down couldn't miss seeing my fluorescent pink running suit. I squeezed between the front bumper of a little red something and the rear bumper of a white van.

I paused, standing beside the white van. Now that I'd figured out how to prevent trashing my ankle, and all I had to worry about was someone turning onto Prince Street, I could get back to replaying my run.

So, what was wrong with my stride? Why wasn't it working the way it should? I stood thinking, my right hand resting toward the rear of the car beside me, where the side curved to horizontal, making the trunk. What wasn't right about my stride yet? Without planning to, I had started rocking forward and back, both feet positioned in a running stride, the way I always started a run—shifting my weight off my right foot forward onto my left. As I rocked, I focused on remembering what running this morning had felt like and what it sounded like. And I tried to imagine what it looked like.

Rushed.

That was it. I felt my gait, felt it rushed. I felt it more like a canter, leading with my right leg, reaching out and then hurrying, trying to catch up with my left. A "canter," except my left leg didn't push off an propelling me onto the right, making my gait rushed and choppy. I kept rocking, just thinking about the image and about what I had to do to change it.

With all my attention intent on understanding what I did when I ran, and on what I should be doing instead, I hadn't noticed the strong February sun that had only just begun rising over the Sacred Heart Church on the other side of North Square, at the beginning of the street, now streaming down toward me, up the length of Prince Street, reflecting in the chrome, the glass, and metal paint lining the right side of the street, to the car I'd rested my hand against. I kept rocking forward and back and thinking: What wasn't I doing that I needed to?

Reaching.

What if I reached out with my left leg, picking it up higher and thrusting it forward, heel down, toe raised?

How could I "cycle" that leg, lunge it out ahead, pushing it forward, pouncing it into the next step? That was what I needed to do, but how?

"If you know what you want to do you can do what you want," I heard Feldenkrais' words reminding me.

Still rocking back and forth while I analyzed what didn't work about my gait, I looked down the solid line of cars stretched out ahead of me along the right side of the one-way street, pulled as close to the gutter as humanly possible, often bumper-to-bumper, front to back actually touching and gleaming at me in the crisp, early-morning winter sun.

On one level, I rocked back and forth just to keep my muscles from tightening up. But at another level, I must have thought What if? Or was it just so obvious that the almost unbroken stretch of parked cars along the right side of the street formed a handrail if I needed it and that the smooth, newly repaved road existed that morning for me to run down?

What was the worst that could happen? I could fall, and any neighbors awake enough to peer out the window might see me . . . So? People had seen me fall before. Besides, after almost ten years, if I wasn't used to picking myself up off public ground, when would I be?

But thoughts of falling, if any entered my mind, didn't register. It was the length of Prince Street that held my attention until I rocked my hips forward, pushing my body weight and momentum over my left foot, initiating the first stride through with my right leg. Go!

Stride after stride, I chanted silently, "Reach-and, reach-and, reach-and, reach-and," the words echoing in my mind until I did speak them, pulling breath in through my nose and then exhaling the "and." Then, long and drawn out, I thought, telling myself, Atta girl, atta girl, and keep goin', keep goin', keep goin'. My right hand I held at chest height, neither brushing a handrail nor against the cars beside me, but rather in a loose fist, my arm pumping with my leg and feeling natural that way.

A car had pulled into the alley-street called La Fayette Avenue, parking there, its rear bumper fitting even with the cars parked on either side of it, giving me a waist-high something to reach for should I need it—though I was doing without. I just kept going, "Reach-and, reach-and, reach-and, reach-and . . . " When I got to the alley beside my building, I found another car had parked across, blocking the entrance. Part of me knew I was running without using the cars, but just in case, it helped to know I could if I needed to.

Thwaack-thwack, thwaack-thwack, thwaack-thwack, my feet pounded the pavement, still unevenly. Thwaack-thwack, thwaack-thwack, the step with my left leg still coming faster than it should and sounding longer. "Reach-and. Reach-and. Reach-and," I was chanting out loud now, trying to time my words to the rhythm my gait should have.

Come-on, come-on, keep-goin', keep-goin', atta girl, I thought to the beat of reach-and, reach-and, reach-and. Already past the alley. Reach-and, reach-and, reach-and. I was doing this!! The realization came to the front of my mind, along with a rush of exhilaration.

Come on girl, you're doing fine, just focus. Focus. Focus. There. More. To the corner. Focus. Focus. Reach-and. Reach-and. Reach-and. As I ran around the hood of the white Bova Bakery delivery van, I glanced down Salem Street to my right—another one-way street. I could just round the corner and keep going. But should I? Should I keep going? Should I keep running? The parked cars lined the wrong side for me and my legs were tired already, and now, more so from running free another quarter mile.

But I was doing it! I was running Free! Should I keep going?

No.

I stopped, climbing up onto the sidewalk in front of the Bakery, and stood still a moment. It was so quiet. No one was out—not even hanging around—it was a twenty-four hour bakery.

But I did it! I'd just run free! I just ran without holding onto a handrail.

Hot damn!

Raising my right fist overhead and my left as high as I could, I did a "Rocky." Right there in the street, hearing the tune in my head. Da-da-daa, da-da daa, da-da-daa, da-da-daa. Do-dedo-de-de-deet-de-de-dee de-dee. And I bounced up and down, my head held high, fists punching the air, dancing and grinning.

I shouted silently to myself, Yeee-ha! It was far too early for real celebration, even as I pranced on the sidewalk.

I *was* going to run the Bonne Bell. By fall. I *would* be able to run those ten kilometers. Or maybe more even. Backtracking, but up on the sidewalk now, I rounded the corner home, pausing a moment on the stoop to stretch my Achilles. Sweat dribbled down along the crevass of my spine. I was soaked under the arms. Just realizing that sent a shiver through. The sun might be warm, but it was February. The air still had a bite.

I pushed open the door to the building, stepping into the quiet inside and dim—compared with the bright outdoors. Everyone must still be asleep. The front door closed behind me, not slamming because I caught it.

Unlocking the door to my apartment, I knew before crossing the threshold what would be inside: the magazine I'd browsed last night open on the coffee table, the pillows on the couch neatly arranged. Junk mail and catalogs I hadn't decided whether to open and thumb through or recycle on the wooden trunk by the door. And WBUR, the National Public Radio affiliate, would be airing "Weekend Edition-Saturday." I left the radio on when I was out, always tuned to WBUR.

Still, even with the radio playing, it was quiet—no one in another room to wake up and roust out of bed to make noise and celebrate with and maybe go out to breakfast with. I could call David, or Karan, or Mom maybe. But no . . . I glanced at my watch: quarter to seven. Still far too early to call anyone, even if all through college and when I'd lived in New York Mom had always called before eight o'clock— back in the days when the time of the call made a difference. She might not be up this early, and Dad wouldn't be.

I'd just start the coffee and jump into the shower. Eventually, people would wake up, and I could call Karan, David, Scott, Carol, Ann, Cale, Doug, or somebody . . . Those lucky people on the West Coast. It'd never be too early to call East and share exciting news . . .

"SO WHAT'S YOUR ROUTE TOMORROW?" DAVID ASKED.

I squeezed the receiver to my ear struggling to hear, he spoke so softly. David seemed so unimpressed about my "running free," as if somehow he'd expected me to have gotten to it a lot sooner.

"Tomorrow?" I asked, surprised by the question. It was months now I'd been running every other day—like clockwork. "Tomorrow's an off day. But Monday, I have no idea. I haven't thought that far ahead. Maybe I'll cross over the Charlestown Bridge."

"And then where? That's not even half a mile."

I shook my head once, jerking it toward the right, hard enough to feel my hair rustle. What was it, not even a couple of hours since I'd run without a handrail for the first time? I hadn't allowed myself to consider these next-step possibilities. For months, since October, I'd been focused on getting strong enough to keep going farther around and around the overpass, to getting my leg used to a running stride and into the idea of running.

Until now, running the Bonne Bell, the race they now called the Tufts 10K for women, had been a light at the end of the tunnel, a long, long-term goal. I was supposed to have the middle all planned and ready?

"Maybe I'll follow the Freedom Trail down past the Constitution and then keep going around by that battleship down there, follow the HarborWalk in and around the wharves, and come back. That should be a good run."

"So what else do you have planned for today?"

I laughed. "The regular Saturday morning rush—Haymarketing, miscellaneous errands. Oh! I'd better get going. I'm also meeting a friend for coffee and breakfast in Harvard Square. Gotta roll, bye." And maybe, I thought to myself, I'll find out when they'd next run the Tufts 10K. For some reason, I thought, in autumn.

After hanging up, still holding the cordless phone, I lowered myself to the floor to stretch again. Hmm, that was funny. My right gluteus was really tender this morning. I stretched, shifting a tad side to side, trying to find where in the muscle I'd strained it. Oo-oo-ww, there it was, and it was definitely tender—not damaged, just worked harder than it was used to, and in the process of stiffening up. I stretched, pushing the tenderness. I needed to work through that muscle . . . couldn't have my right leg giving me trouble. There. Okay, that was better.

I climbed up off the floor, bending forward, reaching my palm to the floor between my feet. Oh, that got it too. Tomorrow I'd walk over to the Navy Yard, down by Old Ironsides, and scout out my Monday morning run.

Twenty:
The Navy Yard

FOR MY SUNDAY MORNING RECONNAISSANCE MISSION in search of a route to run free tomorrow, I wore my old pair of running shoes, recently replaced by new ones and now relegated to walking shoes. The weather had deteriorated from the blue sky and sun of yesterday. It looked and felt like snow coming. Hopefully just a flurry, I thought. Tomorrow I wouldn't be running the meticulously shoveled pedestrian overpass. On the city streets, only dirty remnants of snow remained from the last storm, with a random patch here and there pressed tight against buildings.

Aware now of how I was walking, I noticed my gait seemed stronger, more confident. More even, too? And it sounded better—not so much of my left foot slapping, more of my heel landing first, then the middle of my foot, followed by my toes. My left foot almost seemed to be rolling through the step—and as though I trusted myself to stand on my left leg alone, as long as a step should take, rather than rushing through to the safety of my right leg. My stride seemed longer again today. I smiled to myself, noticing this unanticipated running dividend.

Just across the street ahead was the corner where yesterday I'd stood thinking about my morning run around the walkway, never imagining then that today I'd be looking for the route to run free tomorrow.

I stepped out into Commercial Street—the two travel lanes and parking lane in each direction a daunting distance to cross usually. But with this new walk, my legs felt long enough to handle it easily—besides, on Sunday morning few cars drove the city.

I kept walking, now on the Charlestown Bridge, still studying how it was doing it. Usually I carried a canvas bag or briefcase over my shoulder whenever I went out. This time my hands were free, my shoulders square to my hips. Was that the difference? not carrying a bag? This morning, walking felt more natural than like the elephant on stiletto heels I usually imagined for myself.

It had been at least a year since I'd last walked over the bridge into Charlestown. Off to my right, Old Ironsides' three masts, still decorated with holiday lights, stood taller than the Tudor Wharf building, the remains of the Rapids furniture warehouse still collapsing into the harbor. Behind the ship, new red-brick condominium buildings with names like Constitution Quarters, Flagship Wharf, and the Shipyard Townhouses framed her masts. I'd heard about the move to redevelop the Navy Yard but hadn't explored recently.

I crossed the bridge exposed on either side to expanses of water. A sharp wind off the Harbor on one side and off the Charles River on the other encouraged me to walk briskly. I looked around, without dawdling. Under a gray-white overcast New England winter morning sky, the wind off the harbor whipped up choppy waves with a bit of a whitecap.

I could see through to the water as I crossed the steel-grate center span surfacing the full width of the bridge. Tires rolling over the grating beside me sounded different than on asphalt, almost humming. A dropped quarter would plunge through the grid into the harbor, but probably not house keys. How many children walking the Freedom Trail with their parents had squatted down poking fingers through? How would the footing be, running on this, especially in the rain? Would the rubber soles of my sneakers slip, or was the grid small enough to provide traction? One of these days I'd run across in the rain, and then I'd know.

The city maintained the sidewalk on the bridge fairly well, although I had to step around a couple poorly patched holes and over some cracks. I'd have thought it would be perfect, with all the tourists marching over it following the Freedom Trail from the historic sites in the North End to those in Charlestown . . . Oh well, so much for that. I'd just have to watch where I put my feet, learn the holes and cracks, and make sure I didn't turn an ankle.

So this funny dirt path was how people got down to the Constitution, the wharves, and the Navy Yard condos? What a ridiculous challenge for anyone pushing a baby carriage, pulling a suitcase, or wheeling a chair. I hadn't yet tried running on dirt. What would that be like? Would it shift underfoot, maybe make me lose my balance? I supposed it could. But then again, if my foot struck the ground well balanced—side-to-side, as my weight rolled through, wouldn't the dirt allow the toe of my shoe to dig in and push off stronger?

Standing in the dirt path, my feet a stride apart, right ahead of left, I rested my hand, just for balance, on the pole of a sign directing tourists to historic sites. and tried working out what running on dirt would be like. My left toe dug in as I rocked, seeking purchase in the dirt before pushing off. I leaned into the lunge, pressing into my right foot. It was different from cement. Better? Hard to say, since I had no momentum—though maybe it could be. I examined the grainy, sandy, city dirt—not firm-packed loam—and felt the particles shift under my feet, until they seemed to lock together in sort of a ridge. I leaned into my left foot, the heel raised off the ground so it was just my toes bent back and pressing into the earth, trying to get the feel of the dirt underfoot, trying to understand how it acted when stepped on.

I followed the Freedom Trail where it was apparently supposed to go off the dirt path and up onto the sidewalk, until I found the chipped red paint stripe marking the Trail. As I approached the Constitution, I followed the Trail as it alternated between red brick and red paint. Straying from where they wanted visitors to walk led to rough, unrunnable stretches. But still, I left the Trail and walked to the end of the old asphalt-paved wharf jutting into the harbor, between the Constitution and the Cassin Young, a decommissioned World War II destroyer retired to Boston for tourists to see.

They ought to do something with the end of this wharf, I thought. Time and gravity were dragging it into the harbor with all its parking lot debris, including what appeared to be several abandoned cars. And we were spending so much money to clean up Boston Harbor. At the end of the wharf, I stood alone, just looking across and seeing from a different angle the financial district towering over Boston's waterfront, and the landmarks: the Old North Church spire, the Custom House clock tower, the condominiums called Harbor Towers and, in the inland distance, the old Hancock building—its red light flashing steadily, predicting precipitation and the new blue-glass Hancock tower.

Around me, tall, winter-yellowed swamp grass rustled in the breeze, and the other side of the harbor seemed almost close enough to touch. Shivering, I turned to continue walking. It was too cold to stand there looking. Just past the Constitution Museum, I found a finished section of Mayor Flynn's HarborWalk. He'd promised a public access boardwalk that would eventually ring the harbor and bring people walking to the water's edge. I stepped onto the boardwalk. I liked the boardwalk. It was more forgiving to run on.

I glanced at my watch. Just a little more looking around, I thought. David had suggested we get together this afternoon for a movie, and there was so much else that had to be done. But what a wonderful place for running! The air even tasted clean, and, early in the morning, before the tour buses delivered their passengers, the piers would be a private sanctuary in the middle of the city. Running here would be wonderful. If I'd been a kid still, I'd have been jumping up and down. This was why I'd wanted to teach myself to run. Instead, I turned and continued walking. There was more to discover.

Twenty-one:
Crossing into Charlestown

BEEP-BEEP-BEEP. BEEP-BEEP. MONDAY MORNING, FINALLY. Getting to sleep last night was nearly impossible. If *Silence of the Lambs* wasn't enough to keep anyone awake, when I finally shut out the light and pushed Hannibal Lecter out of my mind, all I could think about was running free.

It felt even colder when the alarm went off far too soon. Cold everywhere outside my electric blanket, and dark, really dark. Was it four already? Could I have made a mistake . . .

I could lie there wasting time and wondering, I could roll over and try dialing time and temperature in the dark, or I could assume I set the clock correctly, throw off the covers, and leap out of bed, just as I was supposed to—because, like going for a swim in the cold Atlantic, deciding to and doing without hesitation were the only way to get it done. And what was the point of lying indecisively when today was the day I'd been working toward for so long—the day I really started training to run the Bonne Bell? I threw off the covers.

Passing through the living room, I touched the thermostat. A bit of heat would make stretching go easier and make it less painful to change into my running suit. I rubbed my nose in the palm of my hand to warm it. Already I could hear my jalopy furnace in the basement cranking to blast hot air through the ducts and into my apartment—it wouldn't be long now.

OUTSIDE, STRETCHING MY ACHILLES ON THE STOOP, I watched my breath cloud the air and vaguely contemplated whether I should start running on Prince Street, right in front of the building. Or perhaps, since I was used to walking a ways before launching into a run, should I walk until the beginning of the bridge—sort of warm up my muscles first, get them psyched up.

How did runners usually start? I realized couldn't remember what I'd done before the hemorrhage and the paresis. Probably though—I almost laughed out loud—probably I used to start running right off, since starting slowly and working my way into things would be too sensible and patient, and definitely not my style.

Oh, what the hell. I twisted my head, looking over my

shoulder while I held a good long stretch on that right Achilles. What if I just rocked back and forth, my hand resting against that signpost, and then ran to the intersection? I'd worry about whether I needed to stop to cross over when I got to Commercial Street. The point was to run as long and as far as I could. Too much planning and thinking about how would tense up muscles in my left side, making it impossible. I shifted the stretch onto my left Achilles—umm, yes. That felt good, right through the back of my knee, all the way up my leg. I held the stretch a "ten one-thousand" count."

Both heels hanging over the step edge, I tried something new. I squatted down and, just for balance, still held the handrail with my right hand. Compacted in a ball, my knees touching the stair above, I pressed my heels down, working both calves together. Yes, yes. That was good. But enough stretching—time to just do it. This was going to work.

I rested my hand against the signpost, not wrapping my fingers around. It was for balance, not support. A few back-and-forth rocks, to remind my leg. Maybe someday I wouldn't need the rocking. Maybe someday I'd be able to think "run" and I just would.

I noticed it in the first few steps. Not that it was bad . . . I held both arms bent at the elbow, fingers loosely curled, thrusting my arms forward from the shoulder with each step. This was different from what I'd been doing on the overpass, but it felt right, as if arms were supposed to behave this way. With my right hand always on the handrail, it hadn't been involved in running, only in protecting.

My arms free, pumping away, it almost felt as if they led my stride from the shoulder, helping me shift weight from my right foot onto the left and back . . . As I got closer to the end of the street, I began to consider whether my left arm's pumping was also helping shift weight onto my right foot.

Not enough time. I'd think about that going over the bridge, after I negotiated the intersection. I hated to stop running, but the signal lights, at this hour, flashing yellow in one direction and red in another didn't give anyone right-of-way. Looking up and down the five converging streets, I saw no vehicles headed toward me—only trucks barreling straight over the bridge into Charlestown and those driving Hell-bent-for-leather out of Charlestown off the bridge.

Clearly, quarter to five in the morning was the time to be a pedestrian in "America's Walking City." Having looked, I kept going but paused on the washboard traffic strip to check again before crossing the other half of Commercial Street and onto the bridge.

I didn't notice the views around me—only the ground in front, where I put my feet. With practice, maybe I'd be able to look up and enjoy the harbor beside me. My left arm, still firm at the shoulder, felt surprisingly relaxed at the elbow. Although she didn't hang straight, which wouldn't have been normal running form, nor was she frozen in the sharp, spastic right angle she'd adopted since the hemorrhage. The fingers, though still curled, weren't clenched.

That was different, and I wondered why, especially with

so much activity at the shoulders—the cross-lateral stuff with my arms—my fingers relaxed. Usually the more I tried to do, the tighter my muscles got through the whole left side—but not, it seemed, with running free.

Whoa! Ouch! Umm, nice ankle twist. Hop, hop, hop. Good save, right leg.

Serves me right for not paying attention to what I'm doing. Running free is a lot more to think about than running with a handrail. I rocked side-to-side, my feet shoulder-width apart, working the twist out of my left foot's body memory, out of my ankle's recollection of how things had just gone awry. Rocking side-to-side this way reminded my ankle of its proper range of motion, of how far off center my body weight could be without my ankle rolling, of how it feels at the outermost edges, and of how my foot should adjust to prevent my ankle from rolling.

All right, kids— enough roll recovery. Time to get going. We're at least going down to see the Constitution, and then maybe we'll head home. Just that far wouldn't be as long a run as around and around the Leverett Circle walkway umpteen times, but somehow, it seemed the effort might be about the same. This running free was harder. Once down to the Constitution, we'd see, I told my leg—maybe it wouldn't be enough. But we'd have to get that far to find out.

I reached to the side, my fingertips just touching the steel balustrade-like bridge wall. Between me and the wall an old ten-inch pipe crossed the river, bracketed to the sidewalk. I couldn't have used this wall like the handrail, even if I'd wanted to. Shifting my feet, left foot a pace ahead of the right, I rocked forward and back, getting myself going again. Besides, I hadn't even tried the dirt yet. I laughed to myself, feeling a lot like I had sitting at the way top of the jungle gym not long after Mom had assured Gram, "Oh, she's okay playing in the front yard by herself. With her arm in a cast, she can't climb around and get herself into too much trouble."

Doing what I wasn't supposed to be able to do always had its allure. I pushed off, running again. "Okay, okay," I said to my leg, "atta girl. Keep goin'." The steel grating underfoot at the center of the bridge was weird to run on. I looked down, watching my feet land, still able to see a pace or so ahead. The water below reflected the lights overhead. The footing was solid—not giving at all as each foot landed, which was probably good . . .

I kept going, listening to the tires of the lone car or two hum over the metal grating as they passed. My shoes didn't grip the grating as well as the cement sidewalk. Up on my toes as I was, my shoes wanted to twist to the side. Focus on rolling through the foot evenly, heel to toe, and big toe to little toe. No pushing big toe onto little toe —that would strain my knees. Keep the momentum going evenly, straight through, heel to toe. That's better, that's it, that's it. Okay, this is good, this is good. Now, can it be more even? Can it be as much time on the right foot as the left? Why is there still that hesitation, a pause on the right before the left foot lands?

Here we are, Kids, the dirt path. Not as different as I'd

imagined. Roll through the foot evenly, big toe to little toe, just like on the steel grating. This is pretty nice. Dirt's a softer landing. Of course! That's why they grade tracks with clay. Keep going, keep going, take the curve nice and wide, then onto the sidewalk. That's a girl—let's try to even it out. You're still way too asymmetrical.

"Reach-and, reach-and, reach-and, reach-and," I chanted, like the measured tap-tap, tap-tap of Mrs. Payette's pencil on the wooden edge of the piano during my lessons. I'd tried so hard to match the meter she wanted. I could hear it perfectly, but how to produce it in music when my fingers wouldn't? Somehow, eventually, I'd get it with my feet on the pavement. Probably not today, but someday. Someday I'd get it, and then I'd really have this right.

But God, it felt so good, just this much—the cold air, my own headwind pushing against my cheeks, tickling my ears and nose and cutting my throat, cooling the underside of my tongue that I held curled up to the roof of my mouth to warm each breath, the headwind cooling the rivers of sweat under my arms, down my spine. All of it felt good: the muscle strain everywhere; my arms, my back, my stomach, my legs.

Just behind the old brick building quartering the sailors commissioned to the Constitution was the basin where they tied up the old frigate. Rounding the corner, I found her alone, quietly floating in bathtub-still water, all her lines slack, the white paint on her bow almost iridescent in the dark against her old black oak hull—the hull that had repelled so many British cannonballs aimed to sink her during the Revolution, earning her the nickname "Old Ironsides." So early in the morning, I alone witnessed her, while even her sailors slept. The morning sky framed between her masts was just beginning to lighten and I caught a glimpse, between two of her three masts, of the Old North Church spire—the "One if by land, two if by sea" spire. Just across from her decks were the slate gray, winter-calm harbor and the few remaining winter-moored boats gently rocking.

Now this, I thought as I ran past, is inspirational. "Reach-and, reach-and, reach-and," I chanted under my breath. Overhead, a seagull coasted on an air current, its wings outstretched and legs tucked underneath. In another hour or so it'd be shrieking, as if to make sure anyone below saw how high and how fast it flew. But it was early yet, and the bird flew silently.

I ran alongside the Constitution and around the wharf toward the Cassin Young. This side of the pier was in pretty bad shape—an excellent place to trip on broken asphalt. Farther down was the Courageous Sailing Center Wharf, complete with freshly poured asphalt, at least partway around. "Reach-and, reach-and, reach-and." I thought I'd round the Sailing Center and then, check out what "running free" on the boardwalk was like. Then maybe I'd head for home.

Twenty-two:
The Financial Five

KNOWING ME, I'D GET BORED AND RUNNING WOULD LOSE it's appeal if I allowed it to become routine, iby running only the one route every other day, month after month. It wouldn't matter that ducks paddling in the water beside me, seagulls soaring silently overhead, sunrises, and whatever else on the harbor entertained only a tiny segment of my brain—that fraction not focused on how I did what I did and on doing it better. If what I saw around me stopped stimulating that fraction of my brain, getting up at four in the morning to run would lose its appeal even if my road race, the Tufts 10K, was in sight, just six months away.

I still got my run started each morning by rocking, and though the toe of my left shoe, wasn't catching so much, the sole, still brushed the pavement.

It was work, this getting better at running, new interesting scenery around me might be the stimulation I needed to keep me practicing.

Every now and again, I'd find the fraction of my brain not consumed with the mechanics of running wondering what I looked like running. Odd, I imagined. It must. The few people out that early in the morning who spoke typically would ask, "Are you all right?" "Twist your ankle?" Some even came out and asked, "What's wrong with that leg?" Then, of course, there were still the "inspiration" remarks. Hey, I was just doing what I had to do.

So where else could I run? I wondered, stepping out onto the front stoop. It was Saturday and a perfect day for exploring. Dinner tonight was at my folks', for what I laughingly called the "April Babies Birthday Party." My older brother, sister, and I were all born in April. Since we were kids, there'd been one day and one cake to celebrate. What if I went up and over Snowhill? The street, just off Prince climbed a short but steep hill. What would that be like? I'd only run along the flat so far, except along the gentle, even, graded sections of the the walkway over Leverett Circle.

I stepped off the stoop, my Achilles stretched and ready to run, leaving my hand still on the handrail, and squatted, heels flat on the sidewalk, stretching my calves. It felt like a stretch I needed to add this morning. Crossing Prince I walked the half block to the foot of Snowhill and looked up the close, brick-lined street. I could imagine Mom describing it with a laugh, calling Snowhill "quite a toboggan ride."

Okay, up you go, I thought. A thick stuccoed green column supporting upper stories of the corner building bordered the sidewalk. I reached out, touching the column with my fingertips for balance before beginning my back and forth rocking. Once I got going, I thought I'd just run to the edge and step off the cement sidewalk onto the blacktop at the curb cut, in two strides or less . . . Since I'd begun running free, I'd quickly discovered how much easier asphalt ran than cement, with boardwalk best of all. This early in the morning—and a Saturday—I'd run up the side of the narrow one-way street, not on the cement sidewalk.

It was different, going uphill. The ground seemed to come faster, and my other foot seemed to leave the ground slower. All in all, it seemed each stride took the same amount of time—only the timing felt different. I found my body wanted to run in more of a crouch. To lower my center of balance, because it would be less of a fall? Or maybe because crouching shortened my stride, thus lessening the timing difference.

I worked harder pushing off uphill to drive myself into each next stride. And I felt the extra effort—in my quads and in my buttocks. Oh, everywhere, I felt it in my calves, ankles, toes, and in my lungs. Up and up I pushed, the cllopp-clop of my footsteps seeming louder here as it echoed off brick buildings and the brick wall for the Gassie playground and the brick wall up ahead for the Copps Hill Burial Ground. At the top, I glanced at my watch—that hadn't taken any time at all. Now down to Commercial Street, toward the harbor. I looked to my right, along one-way Charter Street. In the predawn twilight, anyone driving a car would use headlights. No one drove the neighborhood streets in my view.

I started downhill, noticing the difference right away. In

179

just a few strides I found running more crouched seemed to help running downhill too. Downhill was a different weird. How did your weight roll through each foot—heel through arch and then onto toes? Was it my butt hanging out over my heels in the crouch that kept me from following my momentum and gravity into somersaulting down? Maybe . . . It felt infinitely possible, since I wasn't tipping into a somersault down into Commercial Street.

What would it be like if I landed my feet toe to the ground first? Would it be better if I ran "tiptoeing" down hill? Or would it pitch me forward and land me flat out on my face? I couldn't imagine, so I experimented and tried running "tiptoe." After a few steps, I quit, it was just too bizarre, though I kept running, transitioning out of "tiptoe" as much as I could by tightening my crouch.

New, amber-colored street lights lit the intersection at the bottom of the hill almost day-bright, even in the twilight of early morning. But between the pools of light, shadows spilled deep enough that a driver—though there didn't seem to be any out yet—might not see me, even in my pink suit. If I intended to run the streets, I thought as I crossed Commercial, staying on the asphalt and not climbing over the curb onto the cement sidewalk, I needed to wear reflectors. Maybe at Sports Magic, Ted had something I could wear. . .

In not too many steps, I reached the softball field and my granite wall, a place I hadn't been since discovering the Leverett Circle overpass and then the Navy Yard.

It was like going back to the old elementary school. What once seemed immense. . . In just a moment, I'd already run the length of the wall. It hardly seemed possible this could have been my running universe once.

Whoa. Pay attention Tomm. The sole of my left shoe caught, dragging along the pavement. Hop, hop, hop. I bounced on my right leg, catching my balance again without losing much momentum.

Damn, what was that? I'd already started moving forward again, listening carefully to my left foot, now strides past the incident. What was different? It had been different. But what, exactly? Nothing came to mind, so I kept going, focused on running, until I noticed a funny little street that didn't seem to do much of anything except border a restaurant, dead-end at the harbor, and widen into Christopher Columbus Park.

I kept running, along the walkway around the park, remembering it from five years ago as a chain-link fenced-in work zone around a bronze statue set on a too-big granite block pedestal. The park looked better now, but still no vines clung to the legs or crossed the arch of a rough-hewn wooden trellis forming a center edge. I couldn't look too closely at park specifics—my running wasn't there yet—so what I took in were more vague impressions of the obvious, few details. I retraced my steps some, just enough to try running along a sandy path heading off to the side and into the middle of the park, curious to see what the sand would feel like when I ran on it.

It was only a little like the dirt path down to the Navy Yard. The path was level and the more consistent grains felt good underfoot—no pebbles or stones. But my running.— What was different? Why had my left foot caught before?

What was going on just before the sole of my left shoe had scraped the pavement?

Rolling through. I concentrated on my left foot. It wasn't exactly rolling through now. How was it different when it did roll through? I thought about it, remembering. How could I describe how odd rolling through felt? I'd have to do it again.

Not far past the Aquarium was that new Harbor Hotel and its keyhole arch to the harbor. I climbed onto the sidewalk to take a closer look. I'd passed the arch countless times on the way home from work and, riding around the city. But I'd never seen the sundial mosaic floor of the arch. Looking down at my feet, I followed the circle around like a yellow brick road, just because it was there. On one side of me, the elevated Central Artery shadowed an almost deserted Atlantic Avenue. On the other side, the sidewalk opened onto an apron out to the harbor, to gangways and ships. A fiery-red sun rose in the keyhole between the buildings, yet I was only vaguely aware of the sunrise in my periphery. I didn't stop running. I didn't turn full face to the rising sun, the clouds in relief and purpled on the horizon Someday, I promised myself, someday I'd be comfortable enough running that I wouldn't need to hold myself in "just the right position." Someday I'd be able to turn my head as I ran—look to the side, even behind me. But now . . .

Instead of turning to look, I ran along the hotel patio toward the sunrise, then turned around, my back to it, until I ran out from under the arch. There was no traffic coming, the light was with me so I ran across Atlantic and under the elevated Artery not exactly sure what the road looked like across there, but it was about time to start turning around and heading home.

According to my watch, it was nearing half the time I usually took for a run. Once across, I continued along the Surface Artery, beside the Elevated just to my left. My cllopp, clop footsteps echoed in the metal highway overhead.

Turning onto Milk Street, my footsteps seemed to reverberate even louder against the multiple-storied brick and granite buildings lining both sides. Even as the sun rose over the water, its reds, oranges, and yellows staining the horizon, it was still early twilight at street level, though the many streetlights lit my way. I kept running along the side, running in the street.

Predawn Saturday financial-district traffic consisted of a random cab, a delivery truck now and again, and a lone passenger car. Not sure where I'd end up, I kept running. Eventually I'd come to something I recognized. Milk Street was reasonably well-paved. As I ran I passed more oldish brick and granite buildings but also some newish glass ones on either side reflecting my cllopp, clop. My legs still felt good. I could keep going. I was running well enough.

And then, in front of me—Post Office Square Park! I ran the wide brick sidewalk between strips of grass and low plantings on either side, past the glass headhouses for escalators into and out of the parking garage below. I didn't remember it so almost complete. This summer, maybe with flowers, some benches, and whatever the construction in the corner was going to be, it would be truly wonderful here. Now, maybe a couple of times a week I'd run by and follow the progress finishing the park.

Still feeling lost within familiar surroundings I couldn't place, and not sure what would come next, in no time I passed the old State House thinking, Oh, look what I found. . . I continued down what I now knew was Congress Street toward Haymarket Square garage, getting close to the North End. I knew where I was now. Running down the gentle incline, I felt the weirdness again and, without thinking, crouched tighter, the way I had down Snowhill. And I listened to how my left foot was rolling more through my heel to my toes, to why it felt so precarious.

That was it! Feeling it again, I understood the weirdness. Rolling through stretched the sinews throughout my foot, throughout my heel, instep, toes, and side to side throughout the width of my foot. It pulled, tingling, and confusing me, feeling like the Crick and Watson DNA double helix looked. How long had it been since I'd heard that lecture and seen the diagram? Freshman year college? The tingling traveled, spiraling up my calf, into my knee, and further up. A couple times, as I ran the last leg home, still a number of blocks away, the sole of my confused left foot caught against the pavement, tripping me.

Rolling through was the right thing to do, but after all these years of not being able to, it felt peculiar, and the peculiarity changed the dynamics in my left foot and leg. I didn't know how to translate what I felt. It was like overload from sweet, sour, and spicy hot at the same time. Which did you acknowledge first?

But now that I knew, wouldn't that help? As I wondered, my left foot scuffed the pavement again, but it was almost okay. I didn't trip and I didn't hop, hop. I just kept running.

Twenty-three:
The Guy on a Bicycle

I AWOKE TO NEWS ON MY RADIO ALARM WARNING ME ABOUT rain falling in Boston. Before I even opened my eyes to look, I knew it wouldn't be a friendly summer rain pattering against the bedroom window. How could it be? It was late September and fall-like out there. I got up and pulled on a T-shirt. Today was a running day and in a few weeks I was running the Tufts 10K. I hesitated to step into my shorts. I didn't want to be cold, but my pink pants would be impossible to run in wet.

So what choice did I have? I wondered as I scanned the room. My gaze caught on the electric blue of a pair of Lycra stretch pants Karan had given me that I'd never worn and had stuck on the second shelf of my closet. I reached up for them, remembering how naked I'd felt the one time I'd pulled the form-fitting Lycra over my legs. They were like thick nylons. If I wore my T-shirt untucked . . . it hung well below my hips . . . I'd be covered. Besides, who'd be out there looking on a day like today?

I STEPPED OUT FROM UNDER THE AWNING SHELTERING the front stoop and into the intermittent but huge raindrops. Even with my T-shirt hanging long, I still felt exposed in these pants. But I noticed the cold raindrops splattering on my thigh seemed to bead up instead of soaking into the material, and I didn't feel the cold wet on my leg the way I did on my shoulder through my T-shirt.

Running toward the bridge, I thought of how yucky my warm-up suit pants would have felt by now—heavy and rain-soaked. if I'd worn my shorts, the wind whipping as I crossed the bridge would have sent me back home. My painter's-cap visor worked well at keeping the rain out of my eyes.

Maybe I should have run the "Financial Five" this morning, but having grown up on the shorefront, I yearned to watch stormy weather on the water—even this little stormy weather and on secluded Boston Harbor waters. Before I got close to it, I knew the water in the Constitution's basin would be mill-pond smooth and that the two-hundred-year-old warship would be perfectly safe. But maybe farther around it would be interesting, past where boats were winter-moored in the harbor, others tied up at the piers.

Running my route, I saw almost no one was out this morning. and wondered what the dogs did when their owners didn't take them out to do their morning business.

I'D RUN HARD, NOT GOING ANY FASTER THAT I COULD SEE, but I'd worked up a sweat—perhaps because the hat kept in a lot of body heat. Even after almost an hour out there, I wasn't as cold as I'd thought I would be. I wasn't really cold at all, but it was good I was rounding the corner onto the bridge, practically finished with the run. Ahead of me, a couple of people walked across the bridge, struggling with their umbrellas. Even working harder at this run, it must have been slower this morning—I didn't usually see anyone walking to work I glanced at my watch—a few minutes slower. I thought about trying to pick up my pace. The rain had started coming down heavier, and hurrying to get home so I could step into a hot shower was sounding most appealing.

Just past the center of the bridge, where the sidewalk narrowed to accommodate bridge apparatus—had this ever been a drawbridge? I heard the dring-dring of an old-fashioned bicycle bell. Edging closer to the right, I made room for the rider to pass me, hoping my left foot wouldn't scrape on the sidewalk and slow me down. In this weather, that bike had no brakes, and I didn't like the idea of a brakeless bicycle breathing down my back.

Moving far too quickly for the antique he rode, the strange man—I caught only a glimpse of him in his long yellow slicker, rubber globes on his hands—shouted as he passed, "You'd run much faster if you didn't wear such tight pants!"

I nearly tripped, barking out an "Oh!" on an exhale—thinking to myself Is that the problem! And all this time I've been blaming it on a cerebral hemorrhage! Silly me. . .

I left it at that. It was a great laugh and who needed the negative energy from filling him in? Besides this would be a cocktail-party story—or for Thanksgiving! This was why I was running, I laughed to myself. Walking oddly was never this funny.

Twenty-four:
The Tufts 10K

WALL STREET DIDN'T OBSERVE THE COLUMBUS DAY HOLIDAY.
I'd put in for a reluctantly approved elective, day off.

Starting six weeks before the race day, once a weekend all
September and into October, I'd ridden the subway to the
Arlington Street stop and run the Tufts 10K race route. I
already knew I could run the distance. I also knew I could
very well be the last across the finish.10K winners ran the
race in half an hour. But come hell or high water, I was going
to finish. I'd told everyone I was running—friends, family,
even a few people at work. So I had to finish.

The morning dawned beautifully, but the start wasn't until
nine. I stared at the clock: 4:30. Damn. What was I supposed
to do for the next four and a half hours?

Mom and Dad had insisted on driving into Boston to take me to the start. Of course they were going to watch the race! Mom had said. I hadn't expected that. Running had been my thing solo all this time. I knew I didn't run "correctly," and they would notice that. Once upon a time, probably as far back as junior high, I'd run correctly, and they would have to see the difference.

What would it be like at the start? Should I be somewhere off to the side on the left and back, and plan to cross the line after the "real" runners had started? I lay in bed, staring at the ceiling, trying to imagine how it would be at the start. Why had I never seen an aerial camera shot for the start of a road race—the Olympics, the Boston Marathon, the New York Marathon? Always it was a streetside angle or head-on. I couldn't remember ever seeing a shot of the start from above.

I stared at the not-right angles of the ceiling in my bedroom, tracing each with my eyes, knowing the degrees had to add up to 360°. When I'd first seen the room, I'd exclaimed to the real-estate agent and the owner who'd watched silently, "Oh, an acute angle!" They'd both stared at me so oddly, I decided against gushing over the obtuse one . . . Even my dad, when I showed him the place, thought I'd said "a cute angle," like some sort of ditzy dame . . .

Anyway, these were going to be long hours, waiting for the start. Was I supposed to eat before I ran? How could I not? Even though David and I had "carbo-loaded" last night at La Famiglia Giorgio—he'd insisted I eat the entire heaping plate of eggplant parmesan with ziti, enough food for a family of four. I ate most of it—I was hungry this morning.

Sharp early morning hunger pangs meant I'd have to eat before running the Tufts 10K. I made myself lie in bed a while longer, my eyes now tracing the mortar between bricks in the wall outside my window and searching for evidence of sun. I could feel the October crisp even in my bedroom. My heat didn't go on until November, maybe even Thanksgiving. I tucked my cold nose into the bend of my elbow careful not to rustle the covers too much and let the cold air in.

If it were really that cold, maybe I should wear my running suit. But then again, if the sun came out, my pink suit would be too much clothing by ten o'clock, when I should be on Commonwealth Avenue, coming up to Arlington, then up Boylston to the Charles Street finish. But with all the standing around at the start, if I just wore my T-shirt and shorts, the kids would be way too cold.

When the clock finally turned to six-thirty, triggering the radio-alarm, I threw off the covers and stepped into my shorts, pulling my running suit on over my T-shirt and shorts. Mom and Dad would have the car. Just before the start I could peel off the suit and leave it with them, assuming my T-shirt and shorts were enough. I brewed a pot of coffee, fixed a bowl of yogurt with fruit and granola, and ate slowly, watching the clock tick even more slowly.

Finally, at twenty past seven, my bowl rinsed and in the dishwasher, the counter wiped, and everything put away, I flopped down on the floor to stretch. Mom and Dad would be early. Since there'd be no place to park the car, I should be stretching my Achilles on the front stoop when they got here.

I leaned hard into my stretch and tried to breathe butter-flies out of my stomach as my muscles relaxed, lengthening. Walking out the door, I picked my number, the safety pins, my sunglasses, and my keys off the table.

I pinned the number to the front of my T-shirt as I walked down the hall to the front door. Sticking myself, I realized I was nervous. How silly, I thought. I wasn't in contention. My time didn't matter, just that I finished. And why wouldn't I? Why wouldn't I finish? Of course, there'd be people watch-ing, and I could crash. . . I shook my head as I stepped out-side, maybe I could erase that thought, into stunningly bright sunlight. At about twenty to eight the air was crisp still, prob-ably near the forty-five degrees I'd heard on the radio. Whether there was wind, I couldn't tell.

That was enough looking around. Dad would be turning the car off Thacher onto Prince Street any time now, and I was supposed to be stretching until I climbed into the back seat behind Mom. I settled my body weight through my right leg and into my heel hanging over the stair edge. Was it because I'd spent more time up and walking around the apartment this morning before stretching my Achilles that it seemed looser? Would my left, too? I held the stretch longer, counting twenty one-thousand instead of the ten or fifteen I usually counted before shifting over to my left foot. The left wasn't noticeably looser. Apparently walking more before stretching hadn't affected the tightness in my left Achilles. At twenty one-thousand I paused, glancing over my right shoulder, half expecting to see the silver hood of Dad's car coming around the corner, Not yet still.

What if? Wouldn't I get a better stretch if my left foot stayed on the sidewalk and I reached my right up onto the top stair? It felt real nice in my right hamstrings and through my hip. I held the stretch, wondering if I could reach my left foot up to the same stair, so I could get this stretch in my left hamstrings and hip.

It wasn't that hard though my left foot reached up to the step imprecisely, like a marionette leg directed by a trainee, wavering uncertainly before resting on the tread. I gripped the handrail firmly, my right hand and leg providing some direction and stability. Ooo, this stretch had to be part of my running routine. Why hadn't I thought of it before? But could I have done it before?

"HI, HONEY. READY TO GO?"

I twisted my head, looking behind me, immediately recognizing Mom's voice. I hadn't heard the car. Careful, I thought. You don't want to screw up extricating yourself from this position, not in front of Mom and Dad. I leaned forward, raising my right heel, the weight on that foot now squarely on my toes. As if it were nothing, I lifted my left foot off the step, pulling it back and down to the sidewalk.

"Yup," I said, laughing. "I have me, my number," I pulled my jacket away to reveal number 573 pinned to my T-shirt, sneakers on my feet . . ." My voice trailed off. "What else could I need?"

"Okay, get in." Dad had leaned toward the open passenger-side window.

Still holding the handrail, I squatted once, until I nearly sat on my ankles, both heels remaining on the sidewalk.

"We're off." I settled myself into the back seat as Dad eased the car forward and glanced into the rearview mirror at the two cars waiting more or less patiently behind us.

It took longer than I'd thought to drive to the race start. Dad dropped us off in front of the Li'l Peach convenience store while he went to find a place to park.

"TOMMYE!"

I turned, startled. The door to the convenience store was still closing behind her as Carol ran across the sidewalk carrying a bottle of juice.

"You're here!" She threw her arms around me. "I can't believe we found you!"

Leaning forward and down to receive her hug, I looked up to see David push through the same door. So he must be the "we." They must have met up in Cambridge and ridden the subway in together.

"I didn't know you guys were coming!" I exclaimed, thinking this was really neat. "Mom,"—I touched her on the arm—"these are my friends Carol and David." Carol squatted down in front of me and, vintage Carol, began vigorously rubbing my left leg. "Come on, David," she commanded, "do the other leg."

Mom watched. While I just stood there. I didn't know what else to do.

"You two didn't get very far," Dad said. "I found a space just around the corner."

David looked at his watch. "I think we should get Tommye up closer to the start."

Most of the numbered women were stripping off their warm-up suits and milling halfway up Beacon Hill.

"I'll meet you at the start," Carol said, squeezing my arm as we crossed onto Beacon Street. It never occurred to me to ask where she was off to. Carol did stuff like that, and there were so many people . . . For a moment, I wished I'd thought to remind her to come back to my place for celebratory champagne and lasagna after the race. The lasagna was, as Mom called it "frozen stiff as a boot" in the car, hopefully defrosting, but if not, there was always the microwave . . .

We pushed through the throngs—many of them men with strollers and young walking children beside a numbered woman—past the stripe laid down on the street that must be the start. I thought I should be back of the start and close enough to the left curb that no one could be on my left, where I wouldn't see them.

"Dad, is the car close enough that you can just shove this

into it?" I picked at my running suit pant leg. It was still cool, but the sun was warm, and once I got running . . .

He nodded, and I squatted down on the curb, peeling off the jacket, then my shoes. Taking off my shoes was the only way I could get out of the pants . . . I stood up.

"We have a very special runner with us today," I vaguely heard the voice over the loudspeaker announce.

"Listen! Listen." Carol caught up to us, breathless. "Listen! I told them!"

"Runner number 573 is stroke survivor Tommye-K. Mayer. A stroke survivor! Can you believe that? Come on, let's give her a cheer!"

Those who heard, and there seemed to have been quite a few, did cheer. Mom and Dad looked at each other. I could see they still weren't sure about this. They were probably as preoccupied as I was about the crowd of numbered women even back this far from the start.

David clapped me on the shoulder. "Way to go Tommye!" He smiled, repeating "Way to go, Tommye Terrific."

Neither he nor Carol seemed to think there was any way I wouldn't finish this run. Holding my bunched-together running suit, Mom handed Dad the jacket, so she could fold the pants. Dad neatened my jacket, holding it at the collar and smoothing out the wrinkles before folding it and handing it over to Mom.

"We'd better get out of the way," David suggested. "It's

only a few minutes to the start."

I watched Mom, Dad, Carol, and David walk downhill across the grass toward the start, my stomach churning, but only a little. Adrenaline, I thought. Around me, numbered women shuffled forward, pressing us all closer to the start. I stood, not wanting to get too close. The farther back I was the less likely I'd get trampled., but not too far back. Where would have been best?

I'm where I am, I thought as I rocked back and forth. Too late to change now. The gun sounded, and the way in front opened up some, quickly filling in again as everyone around me pushed toward the starting line.

I tried to move forward and find a stride, hoping no one was watching, because I knew I looked really crippled, jerkily rush-stepping downhill toward the line.

Damn. This wasn't the way it was supposed to be, with David and Carol watching, though I hadn't seen them.

I stopped, rocking back and forth, once and then twice, thinking Settle down girl, settle down. This was my race. I let a space clear ahead of me. Who cares when I cross the line? It's my race. And I was going to cross it well.

I strode across, hearing Carol and David's "Go Tommye!" and then a few more voices cheering down the hill.

"Keep it going, keep it going, keep it going," I chanted silently, trying to keep up with the women ahead of me, the few I could still see. Most of the runners were probably already around the corner nearing the next one. I knew the route. Though for the race, the streets were closed to traffic, and we ran on asphalt, not on the cement sidewalks where I'd trained.

I'd learned not to pay attention to the scenery surrounding me, though I did hear those who still lined the road long after the front runners had passed cheering me.

Just as I ran past the "Smoots" Bridge, the Harvard/Mass Ave. Bridge, a crowd of numbered women more than halfway through the race ran toward me on the inbound side of Memorial Drive. Well, I knew I wasn't going to win this— Just keep goin', keep goin'. Run your race. As the first half dozen women passed on my left, some shrieked Yes! Others whooped."Their voices overlapping each other and sending shivers up my spine—and again and again, as the "women energy" shrieks passed like a wave through the lead pack passing by. Like a lyric to the shriek, I heard the words: "Looking good, 573. Looking good! Five-Seven-Three! Keep it up! Keep going! Keep going!"

How could I not finish this race? Women at the water stations jogged up to and alongside me with cups of water they gently passed to me, telling me "looking great!"

At the loop-around before heading back to the "Smoots" Bridge, the police officers had climbed out of their cars and re-stopped traffic, allowing me to cross safely. As I passed, I heard one officer tell another, "This woman is incredible." I laughed calling back over my shoulder, "Nope, she's pigheaded. Just ask Mom."

Crossing the Smoots Bridge, I'd caught up to where the others had passed me, but they were long gone. A breeze whipping up whitecaps on the Charles River below cooled me. I ran the sidewalk because cars already owned the re-opened bridge. Sweat dripped off my hair and trickled down my spine, making the breeze feel ice cold.

In Boston again, I waited at the light to turn onto traffic-clogged Commonwealth Avenue, wishing I ran well enough to enjoy the street closings. This was nuts. I didn't want to breathe in all the exhaust. Clean air was why I ran in the morning. Still, I kept going. In reverse order, I passed the alphabetical cross streets, eagerly anticipating Arlington.

"Hey, Tommye Terrific!"

I looked up, startled, to see David stepping into the street to jog beside me, still wearing his gray dress slacks, dress shirt, a blue sweater vest, and necktie. I glanced down at his feet. Yeah, and his leather dress shoes, too.

"How you doing? You're almost done."

I felt that leap of relief all the way through. I was tiring. Then the pang of disappointment, because there was still a ways to go. This was only the Public Garden up ahead. The finish was at the Common.

"Tired?"

"Don't remind me." I said, managing a smile too. "But I'm going to finish this race." I felt the sole of my left foot catch, brushing the pavement. I'd never tried carrying on conversation while running. I am not going to fall, I told myself.

"Can you not talk to me?" I asked, seeing the hurt look. Oh, damn it. Do I have to worry about hurt feelings here too? Left-and, left-and, I kept chanting silently. "Thanks," I exhaled. "I need to concentrate."

David said nothing more, running with me until we turned onto Arlington Street, where the finish line still stood, waiting for me.

"Go, number 573!" Three still-numbered women ran toward me just as I approached the line. The first woman to reach me thrust a pink rose into my hand, shouting with the other two, "Looking great!"

I crossed the line, still running.

"Look Kate, there's Aunt Tommye!" Recognizing Skip's voice, I looked up, way up, and saw two-year-old Kate perched on my brother's shoulders.

"Yeah, Aunt Tommye!" Skip shouted with her, the two of them clapping their hands and shaking their fists.

Mom pushed around Skip hugging me. "You look exhausted, honey."

Carol clapped, bounding up and down, "You did it! And I think I got some great pictures!"

"Tired?" I laughed, prancing in the street with Carol. "Mom, I'm wired. I did it! Come on everybody, let's celebrate! Champagne toast on Prince Street. Last one there's a rotten egg!"

Twenty-five:
Roadblock

AT ABOUT FOUR O'CLOCK IN THE AFTERNOON, JULY 17, 1992, the day the Tall Ships sailed out of Boston Harbor, and twelve hours after an early morning run around my Charlestown Navy Yard route, my post-stroke running career was interrupted for nearly nine years.

The Tall Ships '92 traffic management ban on nonresident vehicular travel and parking in the North End was still in effect when I stepped into the Hanover Street crosswalk to cross. Alas, an automobile making an illegal "U"-turn drove over my still partially paralyzed left foot—despite running.

It may have been consciously unregistered pain and trauma, the shock of seeing the car tire wrapped over my foot, or deep soft-tissue damage causing the RSD (Reflex

Sympathetic Dystrophy) manifesting as dystonia; or all three together that seized my left side with spastic muscle tone equal to what I knew upon awakening from the cerebral-hemorrhage-induced coma in June 1981.

All I know for sure is that only the determination that got me from sitting in a wheelchair to crossing the finish line at the Tufts 10K, then the Feaster Five, then carrying the Olympic Torch through Boston en route to the Games in Barcelona, dragged my re-hemi-paralyzed body the several blocks home.

Once I looked down and saw the car tire wrapped over my foot I lost the ability to flex and extend my left leg at the knee. From that moment on, when my left foot bore weight, my whole leg shook uncontrollably, wracked with severe clonus—a neurological symptom I'd seen incapacitate other stroke survivors but thadn't suffered after my stroke.

Also immediately following the impact of the car tire, the sole of my foot, throughout the arch, became rigid, the toes clawing in. My ankle, not directly involved with the car, angled over the outside of my foot rolling constantly and my arm mirrored the spastic tone in my leg—returning my fingers to the tightly clenched fist, fingernails digging into the palm of my hand. And my elbow, which since the running had hung extended at an almost normal 160° angle, returned to its post-stroke 90° full-tone flex. And my shoulder again hitched up. In my back, the hemiplegic tone lifted my left scapula away from its comfortable fit riding smoothly over my ribs.

It wasn't pretty, the damage just driving the rear passenger side Volkswagen Jetta tire over my foot caused. It set me back to the earliest stages of rehabilitation, erasing ten long years of struggle to almost "pass for normal."

I couldn't imagine going through another ten years of rehabilitation. I just couldn't imagine starting all over again—especially if I could lose the gains so easily. The imp was silenced. I quit emotionally, physically, and spiritually, and I committed myself to dying. I no longer wanted to live.

While my family and friends agreed that what had happened was horrible, they did not agree with quitting, and I wasn't allowed to. But I was allowed to take more than a year off from life, hospitalized. They allowed me to stop pushing myself so hard.

Nearly two years later, I had the strength to consult medical professionals affiliated with some of the best hospitals and medical schools in the country. "Can't explain it," many responded. "Psychosomatic," others claimed. "It's all in your head." I was told until one doctor proclaimed, "You have Reflex Sympathetic Dystrophy." The RSD diagnosis was good news and bad news. Good news because at least I knew what was wrong, but bad news because "RSD can't be cured or resolved. RSD can only be managed. You'll have this problem the rest of your life."

So I was told. I researched RSD, learning everything I could about the disorder, its causes, and its remedies. I tried all the medications, all the prescribed management modalities, even surgical interventions. Alas, the condition progressed into chronic intermittent pain like nothing I'd ever experienced—I was unable to wear my left shoe more than two hours! And one of the proposed remedies a Lumbar Block with Continuous Infusions of Anesthesia resulted in a chronic constant migraine-like headache.

I finally turned to a doctor practicing Traditional Chinese Medicine who had resolved another completely unrelated but equally hopeless condition. After months and months of drinking foul-tasting herbal formulae prescribed by my TCM doctor, accompanied by my Feldenkrais practices and my PT/OT stretching and strengthening protocol, the incurable chronic RSD pain is easing, and the tone in the left side of my body has begun settling down. I'm still trying to manage— that is—to live with a chronic migraine-like headache. Maybe someday that will be resolved.

Twenty-six:
You say, "No one enjoys four in the morning"

A POEM WRITTEN UPON LEARNING WISLAWA SZYMBORSKA had been named 1997 Nobel Laureate for Literature, and hearing her poem which begins, "No one enjoys four in the morning. Not even the ants . . . "

You say
no one enjoys four in the morning.
Not even the ants.
But once there was I,
Tying a running shoe to my stroke-paralyzed foot,
Then the other, donning a sweatband and reflector vest.
Be it warm and humid, raining, icy, sleeting, snowing.
Still dark, streetlights illuminated my singular way.

At four, city streets were mine—quietly mine alone.
Hearing my footsteps, my irregular clop, cllopp,
Often the only sound until the morning greetings:
Dairy, bakery, newspaper deliverymen—always men,
Cabdrivers, who are usually men, dog walkers, and
Police officers, driving lonely streets while others sleep.
Boston, my city belonging to me at four a.m.
But that was then.
And now is different.
A negligent driver
Over my foot in bright daylight.
And my 4 a.m. runs are no more.
I hobble now, braced, and in pain always.
Perhaps now no one enjoys four in the morning.
But once, there was I.

Tommye-K. Mayer
October 4, 1996

Twenty-seven:
Epilogue:
Striking off Again

I'M NINE YEARS OLDER NOW AND NO LONGER ROLLING OUT OF bed at four in the morning, but I still crave the freedom of the moment that makes running different from walking. I crave the moment that when I ran happened over and over, the moment when every part of me is suspended in air, when I'm airborne, when I'm flying.

In September 1999, I began teaching me to run again. I haven't achieved that exciting moment yet, the airborneness, but I'm working on it and barring another run-in with an irresponsible driver, I'll keep kicking and practicing. There are now even more interesting places to run in the Charlestown Navy Yard. The Constitution, Cassin Young, and Boston's Courageous Sailing Center are still there. But now there's a café/canteen there too and the Tavern on the Water toward the end of Pier five, boats tied up to new finger piers with year-round live-aboards, water shuttles taking people all around the harbor, and more reclaimed piers finished with boardwalk and bordered with restored and rebuilt brick buildings. It's great to be back! The dark years were almost nine too many and far too long. And now I'm looking forward to running the Kona Marathon as a member of the American Stroke Association *"Train to End Stroke"* marathon team. After that maybe I'll participate in the next Tufts 10K and mwhatever other run strikes my fancy.

So come on. Get running. Maybe I'll see you out there running the history of Boston with me! Try the Navy Yard and take in some of my favorites.   There's always my Financial Five past Christopher Columbus Park, the Harbor Hotel Arch, Post Office Square Park, the Old State House, and back into the North End. You could choose to run the Esplanade, even going by the Leverett Circle overpass, all the way out to the "Smoots" Bridge. Or maybe you'll find a new route.

Marathon training took me on a twelve mile run into South Boston around Castle Island Park, around Pleasure Bay and over by UMass, still proud to have hosted the first presidential can didate debate of the 2000 election season. The eighteen mile "long run" had me running to my folks' house to hand-deliver a Mother's Day card.

I'll still be running, without a headset. Won't you try listening to the sounds of your running too?

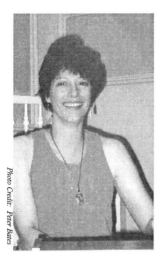

Tommye-Karen Mayer is an experienced speaker, and author of *"One-Handed in a Two-Handed World."* Best described as *"the step-by-step giude to managing just about everything with the use of one hand,* Mayer's book is used in college courses for rehabilitation professional throughout North America.

Mayer may be available to address your organization's next conference. Contact **Prince Gallison Press** at **617-367-5815** to make arrangements.

Mayer has a BA in Sociology from Wheaton College, Norton Massachusetts. One year after graduation she began graduate work in Rehabilitation through the *"School of Hard Knocks"* when she survived a nearly fatal thalamic cerebral hemorrhage. Mayer has been working on rehabilitating herself ever since; Especially after a negligent automobile driver drove over her affected left foot returning her to complete left hemi-paresis ten years after the hemorrhage/stroke.